Defeat Depression

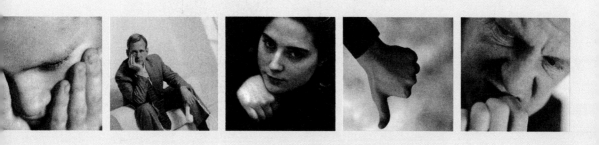

52 Brilliant Ideas

one good idea can change your life

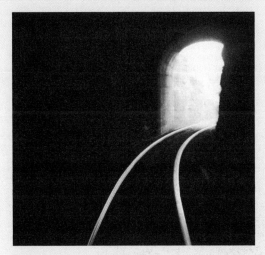

Defeat Depression

Tips and Techniques for Beating the Blues

Sabina Dosani, MD

A Perigee Book

A PERIGEE BOOK
Published by the Penguin Group
Penguin Group (USA) Inc.
375 Hudson Street, New York, New York 10014, USA
Penguin Group (Canada), 90 Eglinton Avenue East, Suite 700, Toronto, Ontario M4P 2Y3, Canada
(a division of Pearson Penguin Canada Inc.)
Penguin Books Ltd., 80 Strand, London WC2R 0RL, England
Penguin Group Ireland, 25 St. Stephen's Green, Dublin 2, Ireland (a division of Penguin Books Ltd.)
Penguin Group (Australia), 250 Camberwell Road, Camberwell, Victoria 3124, Australia
(a division of Pearson Australia Group Pty. Ltd.)
Penguin Books India Pvt. Ltd., 11 Community Centre, Panchsheel Park, New Delhi–110 017, India
Penguin Group (NZ), 67 Apollo Drive, Rosedale, North Shore 0632, New Zealand
(a division of Pearson New Zealand Ltd.)
Penguin Books (South Africa) (Pty.) Ltd., 24 Sturdee Avenue, Rosebank, Johannesburg 2196,
South Africa

Penguin Books Ltd., Registered Offices: 80 Strand, London WC2R 0RL, England

While the author has made every effort to provide accurate telephone numbers and Internet addresses at the time of publication, neither the publisher nor the author assumes any responsibility for errors, or for changes that occur after publication. Further, the publisher does not have any control over and does not assume any responsibility for author or third-party websites or their content.

DEFEAT DEPRESSION

First American edition: October 2007
Originally published in Great Britain in 2005 by The Infinite Ideas Company Limited.

Perigee trade paperback ISBN: 978-0-399-53373-0

PRINTED IN THE UNITED STATES OF AMERICA

10 9 8 7 6 5 4 3 2 1

PUBLISHER'S NOTE: Neither the publisher nor the author is engaged in rendering professional advice or services to the individual reader. The ideas, procedures, and suggestions contained in this book are not intended as a substitute for consulting with your physician. All matters regarding your health require medical supervision. Neither the author nor the publisher shall be liable or responsible for any loss or damage allegedly arising from any information or suggestion in this book.

Most Perigee books are available at special quantity discounts for bulk purchases for sales promotions, premiums, fund-raising, or educational use. Special books, or book excerpts, can also be created to fit specific needs. For details, write: Special Markets, Penguin Group (USA) Inc., 375 Hudson Street, New York, New York 10014.

Brilliant ideas

Brilliant features

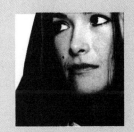

**Each chapter of this book is designed to provide you with an
inspirational idea that you can read quickly and put into practice
right away.**

Throughout you'll find four features that will help you to get right to the
heart of the idea:

- *Try another idea* If this idea looks like a life-changer then there's no time to lose.
  Try another idea will point you straight to a related tip to expand and enhance
  the first.

- *Here's an idea for you* Give it a try—right here, right now—and get an idea of
  how well you're doing so far.

- *Defining ideas* Words of wisdom from masters and mistresses of the art, plus
  some interesting hangers-on.

- *How did it go?* If at first you do succeed try to hide your amazement. If, on the
  other hand, you don't this is where you'll find a Q and A that highlights
  common problems and how to get over them.

Introduction

"God, do I wish that every psychiatrist I have ever dealt with could know what it's like to be a patient and to feel desperate. I wish they could know what it's like to wake up every morning afraid that you're going to live," wrote Elizabeth Wurtzel in *Prozac Nation*. Have you ever felt like that? I have. I might seem like a self-satisfied specialist, peddling depression-defeating ideas, but that's only half the story.

When I was in my third year at medical school, my usual lust for life and energy evaporated. They were replaced by deep sadness and uncharacteristic sluggishness. I thought I could just shake it off. I was wrong. Instead my depression spiraled out of control and seemed to take on a life of its own, robbing me of confidence, cheerfulness, self-esteem and, eventually, my will to live. I felt immensely guilty for things that couldn't have been my fault. Convinced I was a useless burden to other people, I withdrew from friendships and snapped at anyone who tried to cheer me up.

Then, after a botched, halfhearted attempt at suicide, I was admitted to the hospital, where I started discovering some of the ideas in this book. I was incredibly lucky to get what can only be described as Rolls-Royce treatment and learned many depression-busting techniques.

Two months into my admission, I was offered a small sum to take part in a mock exam for doctors specializing in psychiatry. A little cash always comes in handy, so I signed up. A trainee psychiatrist interviewed me for an hour and I hated every minute. He was overconfident, discourteous, and condescending. I thought, *Hey, I'm sure I could do better.* One thing led to another.

When I went back to medical school, and later, working as an intern, I was surprised at how little good-quality information is out there. It seems you can either buy a dumbed-down depression treatment manual written for doctors but translated for the (ahem) nonspecialist, or invest in a doctor-bashing tale of woe by a so-called survivor of the mental health system. I'm delighted that this book helped me do something about it. No miserable stories or miracle cures here, just lots of good ideas.

If the drugs don't work—and let's face it, they sometimes don't—these ideas might.

When it comes to theory, I'm extremely promiscuous. Many of these ideas come from rival schools of therapy. Tips from the mainstream sit alongside techniques from the fringes. If it works, I've added it to my depression-fighting arsenal. The result is a book of straightforward, accessible ideas I can vouch for. I know these 52 ideas work and will work for other people, too. People like you. That doesn't necessarily mean I've been on the receiving end of every one (I'm not that old). Just that I've either tried them on myself or have seen them work with patients. But there isn't anything in this book I wouldn't try.

Despite all good intentions, a doctor's vocabulary invariably becomes littered with jargon. I hope it hasn't crept into my writing. I didn't want to make this book so technical that it was inaccessible, but at a time when many people are taking antidepressants, it would have been crazy not to include a bit about them and an Idea about how our brains work.

My biggest fear in writing this book was that I'd sound like one of those talk show hosts who gush about having "felt your pain." Although depression is common (one in five women and one in ten men suffer from depression), everyone's depression is different; I don't know exactly how you feel, so I won't pretend to. Although some of these ideas look deceptively simple, I know defeating depression is often a long haul. If you've picked up this book, you'll know life can be bumpy sometimes. I hope this book helps you enjoy rather than endure the ride.

That said, like a faithful old friend, depression still pays me a visit from time to time. The dark, dank, dreary winter days usually herald a brief appearance. I've learned how to make it feel unwelcome and show it the door, but I didn't learn this overnight and am still occasionally caught unawares. Fortunately, depression hasn't stopped me from doing anything I've set my mind to. It's undoubtedly made me more empathetic, compassionate, and introspective. I wish I'd understood ten years ago that depression is treatable. If you can believe that during your bleakest moments, you're more than halfway there.

I'm grateful to the many patients, friends, and colleagues who have shared suggestions and ideas for defeating depression. I'm also indebted to Dr. Bernie Rosen, first-rate psychiatrist and top role model. My parents' unrelenting optimism ought to have been ground down by my dark moods. I'm thankful that it wasn't. And finally, thank you, Peter, my husband, best friend, and frontline editor, for bringing more happiness than I could have hoped for or imagined.

1
Look to the stars

Sometimes you just need inspiration. Look to the stars and pick up encouragement and advice from prominent people who overcame depression.

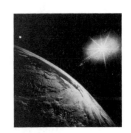

Your own success story might be kick-started by these star-studded suggestions.

Disheartened and dejected? You're in good company. Illustrious names like Charles Dickens, Irving Berlin, Leo Tolstoy, Gustav Mahler, Dorothy Parker, Georgia O'Keeffe, and Michelangelo have all suffered from depression. Composer Sergei Rachmaninov wrote his second piano concerto as a thank-you to the psychiatrist who got him through bad depression. Emulate stars who've overcome depression and you'll acquire some of their strength and temperament. When everything feels like too much of a struggle, borrow some of their determination. Steal some ideas from those who've been to the depths but still made it to the top.

GIVING DEPRESSION A PET NAME: SIR WINSTON CHURCHILL

Fed up with being dismissed as powerless or weak? Winston Churchill was the antithesis of this stereotype. Here's how Dr. Anthony Storr, psychiatrist and author of *Churchill's Black Dog*, described him: "What England needed was not a shrewd, equable, balanced leader. She needed a prophet, a heroic visionary, a man who could dream dreams of victory when all seemed lost. Winston Churchill was such a man; and his inspirational quality owed its dynamic force to the romantic world of fantasy in which he had his true being."

Find your own role model to help you get through tough times. Film stars, pop singers, writers, and Olympic athletes have successfully overcome depression. Find someone who motivates and inspires you and seek out accounts of how they've coped. You might want to copy a few famous lines into your diary, to keep you going when you feel sad and alone.

Yet Churchill was beleaguered by bouts of depression, which he named his "black dog." His pet name stopped him from becoming depressed about being depressed. Dogs are loyal, yet can be trained. They might misbehave and bite but can be overpowered and put down. I hardly need tell you depressed people often blame themselves, but by giving your depression a pet name or personality, you'll realize that you're not the problem, your depression is the problem. Instead of Churchill thinking about himself as a depressed person, he was able to ask himself questions like, "How is the black dog affecting me?" and "Where can I go to get rid of the black dog as quickly as possible?"

HELPING OTHERS: PRINCESS DIANA

After giving birth to a son and heir, William, Diana, Princess of Wales, suffered from postpartum depression. In her infamous *Panorama* TV interview, she recalled, "feeling you didn't want to get out of bed, you felt misunderstood, and just very, very low in yourself. Friends, on my husband's side, were indicating I was unstable, sick, and should be put in a home of some sort in order to get better. I was almost an embarrassment." Initially, Diana coped badly by cutting her arms and legs and binge eating, but then learned to channel her sadness into charitable work, bringing happiness, glamour, and oomph back into her life and the

"I have no spur
To prick the sides of my intent, but only
Vaulting ambition, which o'er-leaps itself
And falls on the other."
WILLIAM SHAKESPEARE, *Macbeth*

lives of others. "I've had difficulties, as everybody has witnessed over the years, but let's now use the knowledge I've gathered to help other people in distress. I think the British people need someone in public life to give

Bored of biography? Turn to IDEA 31, *A novel idea*, to find out how fiction can help you beat depression.

Try another idea...

affection, to make them feel important, to support them, to give them light in their dark tunnels."

SOMETHING TO BELIEVE IN: LEO TOLSTOY

"There is no happiness in life, only occasional flares of it," lamented Leo Tolstoy, who became depressed after completing his epic novel *Anna Karenina*. His life felt meaningless and he became suicidal. At the depths of his despair, Tolstoy found new meaning in Christianity and recovered from his dark moods. I'm not saying you need to go to a church, mosque, or synagogue before you can feel better; just that having something to believe in sometimes helps.

EXPERT HELP CAN CHANGE YOUR LIFE: EDVARD MUNCH

"All I want to do is graduate from high school, go to Europe, marry Christian Slater, and die!"
BUFFY, The Vampire Slayer

Defining idea...

The artist Edvard Munch was deeply depressed during much of his life. Then, in midlife, he asked to be admitted to a psychiatric hospital, spending eight months in a sanatorium. While his early work like *The Scream, The Kiss,* and *The Madonna* is dark and tortured—some critics say these paintings reveal scars left by a miserable childhood—the work he produced after inpatient treatment is different. Elizabeth Cross, a curator of Munch's work, describes it like this: "His introspection is tempered with a love of life, evident in the rich, decorative, Matisse-like quality of his model paintings." There's no doubt about it, they're filled with joy and hope.

How did
it go?

Q **I have nothing in common with celebrities. How could I learn anything from them?**

A *Celebs who've overcome depression and made it are great role models for overcoming this stigmatized condition. Just as you don't need to be like these famous people to admire their music, art, or writing, you don't need a designer lifestyle to copy their ways of coping. Have you ever followed celebrity fashion or diets, copied their hairstyles, or hankered after the secret of those attractive cheekbones? If not, why not seek out mentors closer to home? Others like you have found inspiration in schoolteachers, religious leaders, and neighbors who have successfully beaten melancholy.*

Q **I really admire Kurt Cobain, Sylvia Plath, and Virginia Woolf. Like me, they all had depression, but since they all killed themselves, it doesn't give me a lot of hope. What do you think?**

A *When you're down, it's natural to seek out similar company. This often extends to our musical, artistic, and reading choices. When I was depressed, I read Shakespearian tragedies, Plath's The Bell Jar, and a lot of war poetry. I recognized the emotion, and found it comforting, but I don't think it helped me move forward. I can understand you empathizing with these three, and others like them who've had talented yet tragic lives, but it doesn't mean they're good role models. By all means enjoy their work, but find others to look up to, learn from, and imitate.*

2

Ever-decreasing circles

Depressed about being depressed? Understand what drives your vicious cycle of depression and you'll see how to put the brakes on.

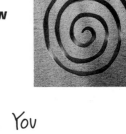

Sometimes there doesn't seem to be a way out of everyday grinds and setbacks. You spend your time reacting to crises. Here are some suggestions to help you get back in charge.

Simon works as a carpenter. He's been married to Katie for twenty-five years and they have two grown sons. Simon is depressed. He's bored at work and when he gets home he can't be bothered to help around the house. So he doesn't. He feels guilty about being depressed. Simon believes he's a good-for-nothing slob. So he behaves like one, lounging in front of the sports channel every night, drinking beer and expecting Katie to wait on him. He thinks Katie is too good for him and stops paying any attention to her. She gets fed up with him and starts nagging. This makes him feel worse so he withdraws and drinks even more, to drown his sorrows. Simon becomes a barfly. His friends avoid him. He's desperate and suicidal. What do you think of Simon? Is he unlucky or could he have prevented some of this? More importantly, what could Simon, his family, or friends do to turn things around?

Here's an idea for you... **Identify one of the things you're doing that keeps your cycle of depression going, then find a way of doing the opposite.**

Try another idea... **Do you wish you could replace unhelpful activities with ones that help you get better? Even your most entrenched behaviors can change if you follow the five-point plan in IDEA 35, *Doin' it differently*.**

DARK GLASSES

Simon, like everyone else with depression, is seeing everything through a pair of dark-tinted glasses.

Any of these sound familiar?

- Everything I do goes wrong.
- She only invited me to dinner because she feels obliged.
- Nothing ever changes so what's the point of trying?
- I only got that job because I was lucky.

Have you noticed that your past is full of gloomy memories and grievances? This happened to Simon, too. Old losses haunted him again and that failed driving test twenty years ago took on new significance. He felt it was proof he's a failure. Perhaps you're also minimizing the things you do well or discounting major achievements as flukes or good luck.

Once the dark glasses are on, it's hard to see other people's views. The beliefs we have about ourselves lead to depressed feelings and this affects what we do.

At the bottom of the cycle is the "action zone." These are some things Simon's doing. You've probably already noticed that they're leading to him feeling even lower, creating a cycle of worsening depression.

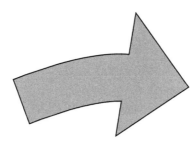

Feelings
Simon feels depressed, tired, doesn't enjoy anything, loses motivation, and has low self-esteem.

Beliefs
Simon's "dark glasses" lead him to believe he's a worthless, useless waste who doesn't deserve friends, family, or a nice house.

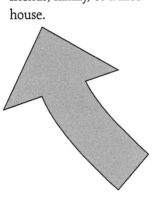

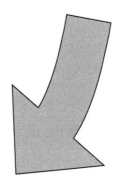

Action zone
Withdrawing at home
↓
Alcohol problems
↓
Losing job and friends
↓
Debt and marital breakdown

If you've been depressed for some time, chances are you've been trying to numb those dreadful feelings. Most people do this by doing things differently. But all too often the things we start doing to feel better end up driving a cycle like Simon's.

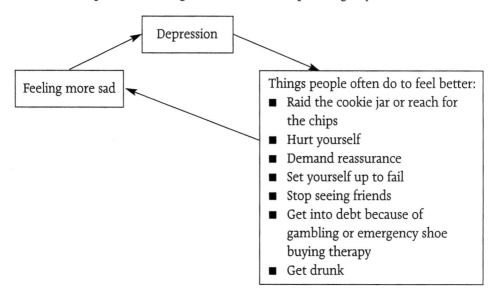

PUTTING A SPOKE IN THE CYCLE

If this cycle seems familiar, it might seem not only accurate but also unchangeable. It isn't. Cycles like this can and ought to be broken. How?

Let's look at what perked Simon up. First, he started teaching carpentry at evening classes. It got him out of the bar, brought in some extra money, helped him feel good about himself, and banished boredom.

Next, he spent some of his teaching money taking Katie away for a weekend and when they got back, he put in a new bathroom for one of his children. He's good at home repair and then didn't feel so bad for shirking the dishes. He's still overweight and would sometimes rather watch TV than go out to work, but he's not depressed anymore.

"A happy person is not a person in a certain set of circumstances, but rather a person with a certain set of attitudes."
HUGH DOWNS, TV host

Defining idea...

Here's how you can put a spoke in your cycle:

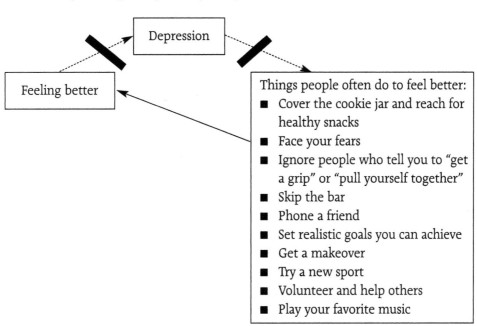

Depression

Feeling better

Things people often do to feel better:
- Cover the cookie jar and reach for healthy snacks
- Face your fears
- Ignore people who tell you to "get a grip" or "pull yourself together"
- Skip the bar
- Phone a friend
- Set realistic goals you can achieve
- Get a makeover
- Try a new sport
- Volunteer and help others
- Play your favorite music

How did
it go?

Q **Every time I try to break my cycle of despair, Mother Nature does something to throw me over the handlebars. Isn't it better I just freewheel?**

A *Life has a habit of throwing obstacles into our paths. The way I see it, these stumbling blocks don't make us depressed, but the way we respond to them can, and often does. Taking small steps to break a cycle of depression means future hurdles won't send you flying.*

Q **I am trying to change my coping strategies but it feels as if I'm just swapping one set of problems for another. I recently gave up smoking, but now I'm eating sweets. Where am I going wrong?**

A *Thinking of every alternative coping mechanism as a potential spoke may mean you end up with the scenario you're describing. But let's not underestimate what you've done. Giving up smoking is a massive step and snacking on a few sweets while you get back to your usual self is the lesser of two evils by a long shot. Now try to think about switching to some healthier snacks, or perhaps some light exercise to get you out of the house and enable you to get some fresh air into your newly cleansed lungs.*

3

Docs, shrinks, and quacks

Dicey doctor or helpful healer? Lots of people claim they'll help you defeat depression. But what do all those letters mean and what can these guys do for you?

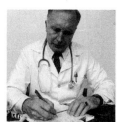

Qualifications can be confusing. How can you know if MD means your doctor has a degree from an accredited college of psychiatry or a piece of paper from a mail-order school?

MEDICAL BREAKDOWN

Psychiatrists: There's a lot of garbage written about psychiatrists. Many people worry they'll be forced to lie on a couch, interpret ink blots, and talk about their mother fixation. This is blatantly untrue. A psychiatrist is a doctor with a degree in medicine and postgraduate training in detecting, diagnosing, and treating mental, emotional, and behavioral disorders. We're also able to prescribe medication.

Here's an idea for you...

Ask your practitioner how much she charges per session. Is there a sliding scale, according to income? Don't be intimidated to talk about the money. Check your health insurance policy or find out if your employer will foot the bill. Will you be expected to hand over a check at the end of each session or will you be billed, and what happens when you miss a session or go on vacation?

Letters to look for:

- PhD: Doctor of Philosophy in Psychology (research degree)
- PsyD: Doctor of Psychology (professional degree)
- MD: Doctor of Medicine—Psychiatry (clinical degree)
- MA: Master of Arts, Psychology
- MS: Master of Science, Psychology

Psychiatric nurses: All-around good guys. These are qualified nurses with specialist training, skills, and knowledge in treating mental, emotional, and behavioral disorders. As well as administering medication, many nurses are trained in one or more talking treatments.

Letters to look for:
- RN (registered nurse)

Psychotherapists: Psychotherapists use talking to assuage depression and explore feelings and relationships. By helping you understand the roots of your depression, they guide you toward recovery. You'll usually meet weekly, same time, same place, for fifty minutes. Unfortunately, anyone can call themselves a psychotherapist, but bona fide ones are members of a professional overseeing body.

Clinical psychologists: Clinical psychologists have an honors degree in psychology and further postgraduate study. Their job usually involves testing and therapy based on the belief that damaging behaviors can be unlearned and unhelpful thoughts can be changed. Psychologists cannot prescribe drugs.

Letters to look for:
- BSc
- PhD

Different professionals have different perspectives on depression. Find out who thinks what in IDEA 25, *Schools of thought.*

Try another idea...

Psychoanalysts: These are the guys with the couches. Up to three times a week, you'll be asked to lie down and talk about your life, relationships, childhood experiences, and dreams.

Social workers: Social workers help you with issues arising from coping with depression or hospitalization. They can help with employment, housing, legal, and financial problems.

Letters to look for:
- MSW (Master of Social Work)
- LISW (Licensed Independent Social Worker)
- LPC (Licensed Professional Counselor)

Occupational therapists: Forget the nasty stories about basket weaving. These trained professionals use work and leisure activities and relaxation to help you develop or regain skills fundamental to overcoming depression. They may have the silliest job title but the substance of their work more than makes up for it.

"He is always saying he is some sort of nerve specialist because it sounds better but everyone knows he is just some sort of janitor in a looney bin."
P. G. WODEHOUSE

Defining idea...

GETTING STARTED

Your first session should be an assessment. Ask yourself, do I feel confident and at ease seeing this person? Beware of the overwhelmingly glitzy or the underwhelmingly impersonal.

Preparing for your first session by making a list of symptoms can be invaluable and helps plan treatment. Try using the following list as a guide, but don't feel you have to leave out symptoms just because they're not on this list:

- Feeling sad (yes, I know it sounds obvious, but you may need to spell it out)
- You no longer enjoy doing things you used to enjoy
- Being tired all the time
- Unexplained aches and pains
- Sleep problems
- Loss of appetite or weight loss
- Loss of interest in sex
- Not being able to do as much as before
- Reduced concentration and attention
- Feeling bad about yourself
- Losing confidence
- Feeling guilty
- Bleak and pessimistic views of the future
- Any thoughts you have had about self-harm or suicide

At the end of your assessment, get answers to these questions:

■ How many times do you think I'll need to see you?
■ How long will my appointments be?
■ What type of treatment do you offer?
■ How long does this treatment take?
■ Am I able to contact you between appointments and how can I get in touch? A behavioral psychologist may encourage email feedback, while some psychotherapists discourage phone contact between sessions.

How did it go?

Q **My occupational health department has referred me to a person-centered counselor. What's the difference between a counselor and a psychotherapist?**

A   *Counseling helps with specific problems or a crisis. Person-centered counseling is an opportunity to talk about how you feel about yourself, other people in your life, and things that have affected you. Psychotherapists tend to focus on childhood experiences, dreams, your unconscious mind, and the dynamics of your relationship with them. But there's no unambiguous difference and the names are used interchangeably. As a general rule, counselors employed in schools, voluntary agencies, or your workplace help people manage everyday problems, like divorce and work stress, rather than severe mental illness. That is often referred to psychotherapists, but there are many exceptions.*

Q **I'd like to see a psychiatrist but don't know how to arrange this. There are so many in the phone book and I can't decide between them. What's the best way?**

A   *Your general practitioner should be your first port of call, as they act as gatekeepers to medical specialists. Ask for recommendations from general practitioners or support groups for people with depression. You could also call community mental health clinics asking how to get referred. If you can't find a clinic, ask your nearest hospital psychiatry department.*

4

Dear diary

Want to try some therapy that's free, versatile, and there whenever you need it? Writing a diary is not just for lovelorn teenagers or third-rate politicians. Here's how to write wrongs.

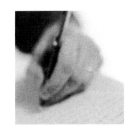

Pausing to record things brings peace and serenity into troubled hearts and lives. Discover what really matters: what grieves you and what brings you joy.

Keeping a daily diary of important events, thoughts, observations, fears, disappointments, hopes, memories, and distress can reduce anxiety, assuage sorrows, and help you defeat depression.

WRITE THE GOOD FIGHT

Aimless ranting? Far from it. As well as putting problems on paper, keeping a diary can help you find answers for stuck or recurring problems. A diary is much more than a friend to confide in. Used effectively, diaries are supporters and collaborators in the struggle against depression. After a few weeks you'll start to notice patterns. Some times of the week or parts of your life make you happy and they'll stick out.

Here's an idea for you... **Put this book down, grab a pen and paper or sit at your computer, and spend twenty minutes writing about how you feel.**

Once you've realized what they are, doing more of them is a fail-safe remedy. Of course, problems and worries can also seem more real once they're on paper, but this doesn't have to be a bad thing. At least you'll know who the enemy is and what you need to work on. Over the months, your diary will be a great mood barometer, and you'll be able to use it to track your recovery and predict what you need to do to get through future tough times.

MELANCHOLIC MEMOIRS

Writing creates a bit of distance that helps you be much more objective about experiences and how they make you think and feel. A nurse I used to work with called diary writing a "psychic enema." Using your diary as a dumping ground for resentment or depression saves you from feeling guilty about unloading on friends. The great thing about putting your thoughts on paper is that you can really be yourself. We all censor ourselves when talking to friends or other helpers, but when it's just you and your journal, you can really let it rip. Notebooks don't hold it against you if you bleat like a selfish, attention-demanding diva. And where else do you get to turn over a new leaf and make a fresh start every day?

Defining idea... *"The truth is that writing is the profound pleasure and being read the superficial."* VIRGINIA WOOLF, depression sufferer and author of *A Writer's Diary*

SPELL IT OUT

Lost for words? Be inspired by some of the great writers in **IDEA 31, *A novel idea*.**

Try another idea...

Writing daily gives you a routine and structure, essentials for beating depression. Try to write at the same time of day, as this gets momentum going and wards off inertia in other areas of your life, too. You know how your moods vary during the day, so you know the best time to write. Mornings work for me, but if you regularly wake up at lunchtime feeling awful, mornings are clearly out. Some people like to create a soothing writing corner with scented candles. Others prefer perching on the end of their bed with a chewed pencil and spiral notebook. I think the key is to find somewhere you can sit comfortably and be relatively uninterrupted.

WRITE AWAY

Getting started is easy. All you need is something to write in (and a pen, of course!). That said, those page-per-view appointment diaries just don't cut it. A page per day is the absolute minimum, but why not opt for a loose-leaf binder? You can add pages or clippings and turn it into a valuable coping resource. Alternatively, going for the deluxe option and splurging makes writing a more sensual experience. Invest in a monogrammed leather journal or embroidered velvet notebook and enjoy filling those thick vellum pages with gorgeous colored inks. Whatever style of diary you go for, reflecting on your day and capturing your feelings is a great way to get started.

"I can shake off everything if I write; my sorrows disappear, my courage is reborn."
ANNE FRANK

Defining idea...

How did
it go?

Q I've never been good with words, my spelling's bad, and my writing slopes in different directions. The thought of keeping a diary just brings back all those hang-ups from school. How can this idea work for me?

A *Hold on, you're not trying to win the Nobel Prize. You don't need a shred of writing talent for diary keeping to be helpful. The most important thing is putting your feelings on paper.*

Q I tried keeping a diary years ago but just kept falling behind. Any tips on how I can make sure that doesn't happen again?

A *Loosen up. You're doing this for yourself and your recovery so it doesn't make sense to give yourself a hard time if your diary sits on a shelf for a few weeks. That said, writing with a specific agenda and thinking about how you want to use your diary should keep you scribbling.*

Q I've thought about keeping a blog. Would this work, too?

A *If you're a dedicated keyboard jockey, this might suit you. But do you really want to share your thoughts about your depression with everyone in cyberspace? Instead, why not set up a new email account as your diary, and email your thoughts to this when you have a spare moment at your desk. (Blackberry addicts can even do this on the move.) You can gather the emails together into one document at your leisure. What's more, the act of writing to yourself can give you a new perspective that you might find useful.*

5
Listen up

The right music can move you from browbeaten to bouncy in just three minutes. It's time to find pearls of pop Prozac in your sea of singles.

As filmmakers, advertisers, and ice-cream truck drivers know, playing the right tune can put you in the mood for love, new sneakers, or a chocolate cone with sprinkles. But music can also help your troubled mind.

Music therapy is a powerful psychological treatment that uses instrumental and vocal activities to change moods, explore feelings, promote self-expression, and increase self-esteem. Ten years ago, researchers at Stanford Medical School studied thirty people with depression. The patients were randomly assigned to three groups. The first group received a weekly visit from a music therapist, the second group used music therapy techniques but didn't see a therapist, and the third group didn't have any form of musical intervention. People in the first two groups had significantly better moods and raised self-esteem and these benefits lasted.

LOONEY TUNES?

To reap some benefits of music therapy, you don't need to see a therapist or buy a new album called *Dance Depression Away with Dolphins* or *Wail with Whales*. Chances

Here's an idea for you... **Next time you're feeling stressed, take a "sound bath." Put some music on your sound system, then cozy up close to the speakers. As you listen, imagine your classical harp or hip-hop jazz fusion washing over you, rinsing off stresses and strains.**

...and another idea **Make a compilation tape or download tracks for a personalized mood-busting playlist. That way, whether you're into Motown or mountain dulcimer, you'll always have music to move you when you need a boost.**

are, you can start to heal your mind with whatever's in your CD collection or on your iPod. Unless you're a metalhead: Scientists at the Center for the Study of Suicide in New Jersey found that a predilection for heavy metal was associated with suicidal preoccupations. Might be time to ditch Iron Maiden and Megadeth and borrow your bachelor uncle's Barry Manilow. Whatever strikes a chord, listen in the dark or with your eyes closed, as your hearing will sharpen when you can't see.

If one of the following moods describes how you're feeling, try one (or more) of my musical prescriptions.

Sluggish: If you're having another duvet day with Enya, you might need to switch to Eminem. Music that's fast and furious wakes up your body and brain. Anything that makes you move is perfect. Think '80s aerobics instructor rather than '90s mood music.

To feel more active, alert, and upbeat, pump up the volume of:

Irene Cara, "Flashdance . . . What a Feeling"
Aretha Franklin, "Rock Steady"
Iggy Pop, "Lust for Life"
Björk, "Human Behavior (Underworld Remix)"

Sad: We've all done it: had our hearts broken and spent an evening wallowing and weeping to sugary crooners. Sometimes when you're feeling low, listening to the sort of slow sentimental mush you can cry to helps. Many pros believe that starting with music that matches your mood and then moving on to more happy, clappy sounds is the way to go. First things first; get out the tissues and play:

Nick Drake, "Pink Moon"
Cranberries, "Disappointment"
Blur, "No Distance Left to Run"
The Verve, "The Drugs Don't Work"
The Clash, "I'm Not Down"

Scared: If you're feeling anxious, music with a slow beat will slow your breathing and racing pulse. Don't panic, play:

Brahms, Symphony no. 2

Stuck or stilted: Depression's renowned for stifling creativity. Upbeat instrumental music jump-starts those bits of gray matter devoted to imagination and resourcefulness. Try:

The Dudley Moore Trio, *Jazz Jubilee*
Bach, *Brandenburg Concertos*
Handel, *Water Music*
Vivaldi, *Four Seasons*

Made your own depression-busting tape or iPod compilation? Great, now move to your groove in IDEA 40, Pedal pushers.

Try another idea...

"Why waste money on psychotherapy when you can listen to Bach's B Minor Mass?"
MICHAEL TORKE, composer

Defining idea...

23

Stressed: Slow, gentle compositions help release muscle tension and lower blood pressure. Choose music with a slow rhythm, ideally slower than your heart rate, which will be about seventy beats per minute. One of these should do the trick:

Bach, *Goldberg Variations*
Pachelbel, *Canon in D*

Sleepy but can't sleep: Lying awake, tossing and turning? Sleeping pills are addictive and can make you feel hungover. Try these songs instead:

Paul Young, "Anywhere I Lay My Head"
Radiohead, "Go To Sleep"
Air, "Another Day"
The Beatles, "Golden Slumbers"
Serge Gainsbourg, "Je T'Aime . . . Moi Non Plus"

Q I'm a student in a shared house. One of my housemates is really noisy so it's impossible for me to sit and listen to music as he's always stomping around, moving furniture, cooking noisily, or vacuuming his rug in the room above mine. What can I do?

How did it go?

A *That house ain't big enough for both of you. Perhaps you should think about looking for another house; headphones might help in the meantime and will also drown out his complaints if the rest of you decide to throw him out instead.*

Q I watch a music channel most of the time, but it doesn't make me feel any better. Why's that?

A *It's probably because you're watching rather than listening. Watching so much television may well be making your depression worse. TV has a deleterious effect on kids' self-esteem and moods and there's no reason to think it's different for adults. Time to turn off the TV and select your own tunes.*

Q I've got a favorite piece of music that I often listen to. I know it doesn't do anything for my mood, but it brings back so many memories for me. What should I do?

A *It sounds like you've got yourself a musical security blanket. Lend the CD to a friend ("You must listen to this. It's one of my favorites. Give it back to me sometime."), delete it from your iPod, throw the tape away, and spend a morning browsing a record store for some new stuff.*

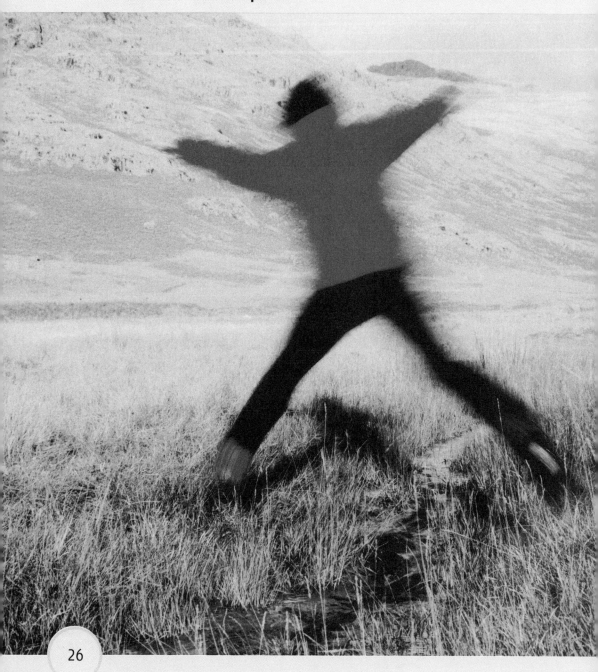

6

A pleasure a day keeps the blues at bay

Dropped the fun stuff? A little bit of what you like does you good. Find out why you need to build some enjoyment into every day.

Depression saps energy and motivation. You're tired, you feel flat, you're fed up, and life just isn't fun anymore. It's hardly surprising you don't feel like doing anything.

Have you stopped going out with friends, dropped out of paragliding, or left your bike rusting in the shed for a second consecutive summer? Is it such a big deal? Frankly, yes, because once you've given up enjoyable activities, you'll start a cycle that'll make you feel worse and you'll end up doing even less.

PLAYING THE BLUES

Sally, a single jazz saxophonist, got the blues after her only son, Chet, left home. Everything took lots of effort. So she stopped playing sax, didn't bother going to friends' gigs, stopped washing her hair, and soon couldn't face answering her phone. Within weeks, she was just doing bare essentials, like ordering in food and turning up her central heating. Sally had no real reason to get out of bed, so she

Here's an idea for you... **Spend ten minutes today doing something you used to really enjoy. It might be returning to a favorite book, playing a much-loved album, or soaking in the tub.**

stayed there for days, thinking about how empty and meaningless life had become. Soon even calling the pizza parlor was too much and she fell into deep depression.

Even if only the first stages of Sally's story sound familiar, it's time to puncture your vicious cycle of inactivity. How? Remember the kind of stuff that used to make your heart soar? No matter if it was kickboxing, karaoke, or knitting, it's time to do it again. When we do things we love, we forget ourselves and lose track of time, and dismal thoughts take a backseat. Doing just one thing that's fun or that gives you that warm glow of achievement will make you feel better. In fact, even planning to do something you enjoy can cause a mini buzz.

Here's how it works:

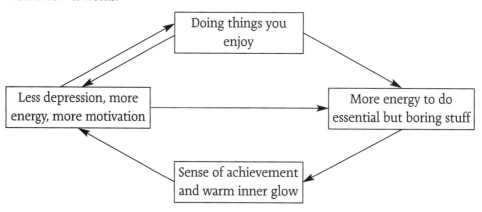

Doing what you enjoy has what pros call a "dose–response effect." This means that the more you do, the better you'll feel. Doing ten nice things a week is twice as good as five. But even one's better than none. It doesn't have to bust your budget or take all afternoon. Here are some ideas to lift black moods:

- Call a friend
- Take a yoga class
- Watch a big sporting event
- Work in the garden
- Borrow a dog and go for a walk
- Dance to a CD
- Watch a funny film
- Get a massage
- Be a lady (or gentleman) who lunches
- Play your kids' video games while they're at school

KEEP IT REAL

Be realistic about what you're going to do:
three rows of knitting before lunch, rather than three striped onesies with matching hats. Mulling over enjoyable times can also hike up your mood. You might like to keep a journal or photo diary to look at when your mood is especially low and use it to spur you on when you feel like staying in bed.

DON'T GO ON A GUILT TRIP

Some people feel guilty about doing fun things when there's a pile of ironing to be done, mouths to feed, reports to write, and deadlines looming. What they don't realize is doing things that are entertaining or exciting helps us do more of those essential but only a teensy-bit-of fun things, like toenail clipping, or oh-so-horrible things nobody likes doing, like taking the trash out. Once you've got your head around this, you'll stop feeling guilty about taking time out for yourself.

Finding it hard to get going? Don't despair: check out IDEA 22, *Actions speak louder than words.*

Try another idea...

"Happiness consists in activity. It is a running stream, not a stagnant pool."
JOHN MASON GOOD, physician and author

Defining idea...

How did
it go?

Q   **I've started reading the newspaper again. It's something I used to really enjoy but now it's having a terrible effect. How can I keep all those sad stories from getting me down?**

A   *It's great that you've been able to revive an old habit. Instead of starting at the news pages, why not read a more lighthearted section like reviews, cartoons, or horoscopes first? Sports fans should beware of bad tidings on the back pages though!*

Q   **I had planned to take my elderly neighbor's dog for a walk, but I've just found out it's been put down. What should I do?**

A   *Oh, dear. Sometimes there are setbacks but they needn't stop you. Instead, try to come up with an alternative. Could you take your neighbor to bingo instead? Cheering her up might help you feel better, too.*

Q   **I loved playing tennis before I got depressed. Then I lost all my get up and go and just sat at home every evening feeling drained and dejected. Recently, I rejoined my tennis club and although it was good to see my old friends, actually playing feels more like a pleasant distraction than the grand passion it used to be. Will I ever feel that good about it again?**

A   *Congratulations on rejoining your tennis club. It's an important step. But try not comparing how you feel after playing tennis to how you used to feel when you weren't depressed. Instead, try comparing how you feel after playing to how you felt a few weeks ago, sitting around doing nothing.*

7

The time of your life

If you're feeling weighed down by tasks like relocating or job hunting, you'll find that good time management is a surefire way to transform your mood and your life.

Whether you want to take a break from the rat race or just want to find the energy to keep up, read on.

Feeling inundated with all those things you need to do? Using to-do lists decreases stress, develops great organizational skills, and improves your memory. Just writing things down means you are 25 percent more likely to do them. Go one better with a daily list that'll show you at a glance what you need to prioritize and what can wait. One method is the ABC list. This list is divided into three sections: A, B, and C. All items placed in section A need to be done today. Items in section B need to be completed within the week. C section items need to be done within the month. As the B or C items become more pertinent, they can be bumped up to the A or B list.

Concentration problems are rife in depression, but a to-do list means you won't forget that hairdresser's appointment or leave your laundry in the machine overnight. Seeing things through to the end is a valuable time-saver, since switching from one task to the next makes you less efficient and more likely to make mistakes. And nothing really beats the sense of achievement you get from crossing off another task.

Here's an idea for you... **Spend a week getting your home spick-and-span and you'll save weeks of time and energy over the coming year. I spent about half an hour a day looking for papers, keys, and lipsticks until I invested in a filing system, key hook, and lipstick holder.**

WHAT'S IT GOING TO TAKE OUT OF YOU?

Get to know your body clock and exploit it. If you're freshest in the early morning, use that time to do difficult tasks like writing a letter to your bank manager fessing up to that unauthorized overdraft. Mechanical jobs like loading the washing machine can be left for when you're feeling brain-dead and worn-out.

HOW TO MANAGE EMAILS

Six billion emails are sent every day, and perhaps you're feeling that most of these are sent to you. If you dread switching on your computer because of the number of messages you'll have to wade through, it's time for action. It's well worth investing in a good spam filter and devising a way of working with emails that need further action. Dragging them into folders for different projects is a simple but effective start. Checking your emails just once or twice a day prevents protracted periods of email ping-pong.

MORNING GLORY

Lots of us are sluggish in the mornings, but you can sneak up to fifteen minutes extra in bed by a little planning the night before. Put cereal (minus milk) into a bowl, fill the coffeemaker, and put out a mug. Take out the next day's clothes. There's nothing worse than getting up and needing to iron, or even wash, a clean shirt.

BIT(E) BY BIT(E)

You probably can't eat a family-size bar of chocolate in one sitting; like most people, you'd break it into smaller, manageable chunks. So chunk up the big stuff and convert those massive jobs into a series of smaller, simpler tasks. For instance, instead of feeling overwhelmed because your house is a mess, set yourself a daily fifteen-minute time frame and work through it room by room. Too low and weary to fill in another job application form? Chunk it up and start with the easy questions you don't need to think about, like your name, address, and date of birth. Once you've got some momentum going, add in things that need more concentration, like your job history. Save any free text sections until you're on a roll.

SNEAKY RUSE

If you're seeing a therapist or doctor, asking for the first appointment of the day or first appointment after their lunch break means you won't be left in the waiting room because they're running late.

Try another idea...

Got so much time on your hands that you're not sure what to do with it? How about a relaxing massage? Check out **IDEA 43, *All hands on deck.***

Defining idea...

"*Time equals Life. Therefore, waste your time and waste your life, or master your time and master your life.*"
ALAN LAKEIN, time-management guru

How did it go?

Q **I work in an open-plan office. Everyone passes my desk since it's next to the kitchen. People stop to chat all day after making drinks and snacks. I don't want to be rude, but all these five-minute chats mount up until I fall behind and end up staying late and coming in early. I feel really frazzled and miserable. What can I do?**

A *I'm tempted to say swap desks with someone, but if that's impossible or impractical, just tell your colleagues you don't have time to talk. If that feels too daunting, try avoiding eye contact when people pass or put up a "please do not disturb" sign.*

Q **I've been avoiding writing my end-of-year dissertation. I just can't get started and have wasted weeks procrastinating. Deadlines are looming. How can I get going?**

A *Instead of thinking of your dissertation as one massive undertaking, try breaking it into smaller sections like research, planning, writing the introduction, writing the main text, and writing the conclusion. Set yourself deadlines for each stage. Setting yourself deadlines might seem counterintuitive, but they give you a series of objectives to work toward. Deadlines will break your deadlock and keep you motivated.*

8

Counting sheep

Quality sleep is a serious depression buster. Here are some reliable routes to regular, refreshing rest.

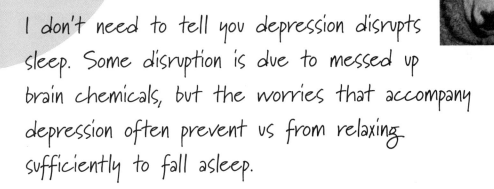

I don't need to tell you depression disrupts sleep. Some disruption is due to messed up brain chemicals, but the worries that accompany depression often prevent us from relaxing sufficiently to fall asleep.

SLEEP SCHEDULES

When I mention bedtime routines, I'm often laughed out of town. I'm not saying you have to be in bed by 7:30 with your PJs on, but it helps to go to sleep and wake up at roughly the same time every day. Evening routines give bodies and minds a chance to wind down. You might like to snuggle up with a good book, play some soothing music, or soak in a warm bath. Light snacks prevent hunger pangs and so can help you sleep better. Heavy, spicy meals are anything but soporific, so skip that vindaloo.

Another good but contradictory tactic is only going to bed if you're tired. If you're not asleep after thirty minutes, get up and only go back when you're sleepy. This can work wonders if you resist the temptation to sneak little daytime naps.

Here's an idea for you...

Once you've set your alarm clock, put it out of sight and avoid checking it if you wake up during the night. Clock-watching can cause insomnia.

UPPERS, DOWNERS, SLEEPERS, WAKERS...

Sleeping pills are addictive and often leave people feeling hungover the next day. They're almost always a bad idea. Melatonin is a supplement that helps some people with insomnia. Our bodies make melatonin, releasing it in increasing amounts from dusk on. If you decide to try it, give it a couple of weeks to see a difference. Valerian is an herbal medicine that some people find helpful.

Tea, coffee, cigarettes, and even that innocent-looking cup of cocoa are stimulants. It's worth cutting these out for two weeks to see if they're culpable. As they're addictive, be prepared for headaches and grumpiness while you withdraw. Warn your loved ones that it's nothing personal.

Perhaps you've found that a stiff drink helps you fall asleep, but are puzzled why you don't feel rested the next day. Alcohol messes up our natural sleep rhythms. When you have a large whisky, you're giving yourself the equivalent of a general anesthetic, knocking yourself out rather than drifting off to the land of Nod. You miss out on the type of sleep you need for that refreshed, lusting-for-life feeling, and when the whisky wears off, you wake up.

Defining idea...

"Sleep is when all the unsorted stuff comes flying out as from a dustbin upset in a high wind."
WILLIAM GOLDING

LIGHT AND HEAT

Falling asleep too early? In the evenings, sit near a bright light to reset your body clock. When it's time for bed, keep your bedroom dark. If you're a shift worker or live in the city, one of those eye masks you get on long-haul flights is just the ticket.

How hot is your bedroom? Most of us sleep better in a cool room, so try leaving a window open or turning down your heat.

Waking up early and in distress? If you're regularly awake more than two hours before your usual waking time, antidepressants may help. Check out IDEA 9, *On the shelf.*

Try another idea...

SHEEP TRICK

If all else fails, count sheep. Visualize them clambering over a gate, one by one. As you start to drop off, your mind might wander and you'll lose count. Never mind, just start again.

A variant is to start with 500 sheep in a pen. Nestle under the covers, close your eyes, and breathe deeply. Every time you breathe out, count a sheep out of the pen. You'll drift off and lose count, but it doesn't matter. The monotony is more important than whether any sheep made a break for it when you weren't looking.

But if none of these tricks has worked for you, rather than lying there worrying about not sleeping, try getting up for half an hour and doing something relaxing before returning to bed. Losing a bit of sleep won't hurt.

"Have you ever had a dream, Neo, that you were so sure was real? What if you were unable to wake from that dream? How would you know the difference between the dream world and the real world?"
THE MATRIX

Defining idea...

How did
it go? **Q** **I've recently had several nightmares where I dream I'm being chased by a shark and can't escape. I see my legs being chewed off. Now I dread going to sleep in case it happens again. What helps?**

A *Poor you. Nightmares are more common when you're upset or anxious. Some pros say our minds make sense of distressing events through nightmares, though how a bad remake of Jaws in the wee hours can help is beyond me. Perversely, going to bed worried about nightmares makes it more likely that you'll have another. Find a compassionate listener and tell them about your shark dream and how it makes you feel. Next, write down your dream in as much detail as you can remember, including all the gruesome details of your leg hanging off. It might sound crazy, but if you read this repeatedly, telling yourself it is just a dream and can't harm you, the nightmares will lose their terrifying power.*

Q **As I drift off to sleep, I can often hear someone calling my name, but there's nobody there. Am I losing it?**

A *No. You're experiencing something called hypnogogic hallucinations. It's not a sign of mental illness; your mind is only playing tricks. Some people experience muscle twitching, or a feeling they're falling or momentarily paralyzed as they fall asleep.*

9

On the shelf

Trillions of antidepressants are prescribed every year. Is there a pill for every ill or are the pros peddling poisons? High time to find out what's in the pharm yard.

Even if you haven't taken drugs for depression, you probably know someone who has. Discover what works, what can make you feel worse, and how to tell the difference.

PILLS FOR ALL ILLS?

Not sure if antidepressants are for you? They're best at busting so-called biological symptoms: changes in sleep pattern, lost appetite, feeling slowed down or agitated, concentration problems, and feeling like your sex drive has driven off somewhere.

It takes up to four weeks for antidepressants to start working. Yep, faster than therapy but tablets won't teach you how to stop thinking depressing thoughts, help you understand why you feel bad, or find a better rate mortgage.

Here's an idea for you... **If you're prone to forgetting your medication, try taping the pill packet to your coffeemaker or teapot. When you make your first drink of the day, you won't be able to forget your pill.**

PHARM YARD

At medical school we were taught to "educate before you medicate," but learning about antidepressants is bewildering. Let's think of them as tribes where members work in similar ways and have comparable side effects. Because each tribe member is slightly different it means if one doesn't help, another from the same tribe might.

Tribe: Tricyclic antidepressants (TCAs)
Members: Amitriptyline, clomipramine, dothiepine, imipramine, trimipramine, lofepramine.
Myth: Old, obsolete, and ought to be left on the shelf.
Reality: Yep, they're an old tribe but they're as effective as any newbie.
Best parts: Can make you feel sleepy so they're great for insomniacs.
Worst parts: Lots of side effects so the dose has to be upped slowly. Can give you a dry mouth, constipation, blurred vision, and drowsiness. Very dangerous in overdose so pros don't give them to suicidal people.

Tribe: Selective serotonin reuptake inhibitors (SSRIs)
Members: Fluoxetine (Prozac), fluvoxamine, paroxetine, sertraline, citalopram.
Myth: Mind-altering, euphoria-inducing party pills that ought to be added to our water supply.
Reality: Choosy about which chemical receptors they'll hook up with so there are few side effects.

Best parts: Won't leave you with a dry mouth or fuzzy head.

Worst parts: Nausea is pretty common in the first few weeks. Can wreak havoc with your love life by delaying your ability to orgasm. Might sound like fun, but gets exasperating.

If you're looking for a cure from Mother Nature rather than daddy drug company, you'll like IDEA 24, *Natural highs*.

Try another idea...

Tribe: Selective noradrenaline reuptake inhibitors (SNRIs)
Member: Reboxetine.
Myth: Newbie sponsored by footwear manufacturers.
Reality: Acts on brain chemical noradrenaline, vital for that perky, zest-for-life feeling.
Best parts: Helps you get going if your motivation's low.
Worst parts: Some people get dry mouth, constipation, drowsiness, and light-headedness.

Tribe: Monoamine oxidase inhibitors (MAOIs)
Members: Phenelzine, selegiline, isocarboxacid.
Myth: Stuffy old tribe with too many rules.
Reality: Oldest antidepressants that were left on the shelf but are now making a comeback because they often work where other tribes have failed.
Best parts: Good for what the trade calls *atypical* depression, a fancy name for comfort eating, oversleeping, being irritable, and feeling hypersensitive.

Defining idea...

"The idea of throwing away my depression, of having to create a whole way of living and being, of having to create a whole new personality that did not contain misery as its leitmotif was daunting. Now, with the help of a biochemical cure, it was going to go away."
ELIZABETH WURTZEL, *Prozac Nation*

Worst parts: Masses of food restrictions. You could suffer a blood pressure hike that can cause a stroke if you eat anything from a long list that includes cheese, anything with yeast (afraid that includes beer), red wine, and pickled herrings. The same reaction happens with many over-the-counter drugs.

Tribe: Reversible inhibitors of monoamine oxidase type A (RIMAs)
Members: Moclobemide.
Myth: Old pills in new packets.
Reality: A better, safer MAOI.
Best parts: Few side effects and no food restrictions.
Worst parts: Insomnia, dizziness, and headaches.

Tribe: Noradrenaline and selective serotonin reuptake inhibitors (NASSAs)
Members: Mirtazepine.
Myth: Antidepressants for astronauts.
Reality: Often refreshes the parts other tribes haven't reached.
Best parts: May have an effect more quickly than other tribes.
Worst parts: Avoid alcohol, as it may make you more sleepy.

Tribe: Dual uptake inhibitor
Members: Venlafaxine, milnacipran.
Myth: TCAs renamed.
Reality: The best of TCAs without their hassles.
Best parts: Works quickly.
Worst parts: Nightmares, loss of interest in sex.

Q   My doctor has suggested I take Nardil. How can I find out which tribe it's in?

How did it go?

A   *I've used generic drug names. Confusingly, all drugs have more than one name. Each has a universal generic name, like phenelzine. Manufacturers give a trade name, like Nardil, which is often different in different countries. This is annoying for everyone except marketing types because it's easier to sell a drug called Damnitall than pleboxyflymoxyethymethylamine. The best-known trade name is Prozac—once the new kid on the antidepressant block, now one of its stars.*

Q   I feel better. Can I stop taking drugs?

A   *Hold on. Before you flush your fluvoxamine down the toilet, I ought to mention that it's a good strategy to keep taking antidepressants even after you feel better. Why? If you stop taking them as soon as you're better, chances are you'll relapse. The odds of this happening are about 60 percent, which is pretty scary. Lots of people think this is because drugs just mask depression and it gets them a lot of bad press. In fact, relapses happen because your brain chemistry is still fuddled. Chemical systems recover slowly. If you continue taking antidepressants for six months after you feel better, your risk of relapsing falls to a measly 10 percent. It's worth hanging in there for six months, showing a little dedication to your medication.*

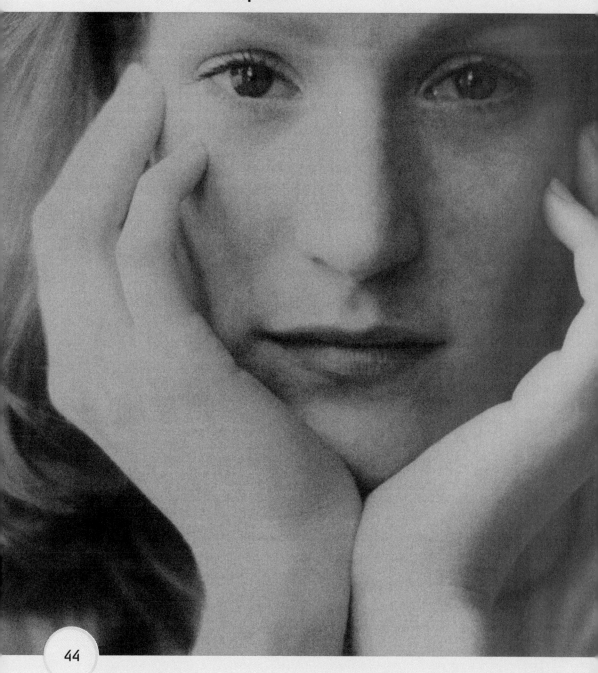

10

Feeling SAD?

For many people, less daylight equals less happiness. Use these illuminating tips to brighten up and avoid another winter of discontent.

Long, dark days getting you down? Sun shortage can cause sadness ranging from dark moods to a condition called Seasonal Affective Disorder, or SAD. Learn how to stop dreading the end of autumn and lighten up.

Everyone seems happier in the summer, and many of us feel more gloomy when it gets grayer. But some people get depressed every winter. A diagnosis of SAD can only be made after three or more consecutive winters of symptoms. If you feel depressed in winter, so-so in autumn, and full of the joys of spring in, um, spring, then you're officially SAD. SAD symptoms are similar to nonseasonal depression but rather than losing weight or waking early, if you've got SAD you're more likely to oversleep and reach for the cookie jar to satisfy carb cravings. People suffer from SAD throughout the northern and southern hemispheres but it is unsurprisingly rare if you live within thirty degrees of the equator, as daylight hours are long and exceptionally bright.

Here's an idea for you...

Plan a "summer" vacation in winter. A couple of weeks of long daylight hours to tide you over until spring may be just what the doctor ordered. Why just dream of a white (sandy beach) Christmas?

LIGHT RELIEF

In northern Sweden there are only a few hours of winter daylight and some days with no light at all. Stockholm psychiatrists got a group of depressed patients together. They split them into two groups: one group who felt depressed in winter and a second group whose depression didn't change with the seasons. All patients were given treatment with a light box for ten days. Patients in the first group (whose depression had a seasonal pattern) got a lot better with light box treatment. But those in the second group, who felt low whatever the weather, didn't improve much with light treatment.

Want some of what they had? Light boxes are readily available. If you buy a light box, use it daily from when your first symptoms appear. You'll need to sit an arm's length away for between 60 and 90 minutes. Sometimes people think they need to stare straight at it, but you don't have to put your life on hold like that. Let's face it, who's got time? You can read, mark student essays, eat, perfect your macramé; in fact, anything you like as long as you're reasonably stationary. Many people, feel better after three or four days but that wears off unless it's used every day. 'Nuff said.

COULD YOU DO WITH A D?

Scientists have discovered that vitamin D supplements help SAD sufferers. They thought vitamin D deficiency might play a role in SAD.

No great surprise, since it's been called "the sunshine vitamin." Ultraviolet rays from sunlight react on your skin, producing a form of vitamin D. People with SAD who took a vitamin D supplement every day for five days noticed a lift in their winter blues. They took 400 IU of vitamin D. Guess how much a teaspoon of cod liver oil contains? 400 IU.

I've yet to meet anyone who likes the taste of cod liver oil, so if you've wrinkled your nose, you're in good company and might like to try shrimp, sardines, mackerel, or salmon instead—these foods are rich in vitamin D. If you're a vegetarian you'll get small amounts of vitamin D from creamy milk and egg yolks. If you've gone the whole hog (so to speak) and are vegan, you'll need to eat fortified foods—like soy milk, margarine, and breakfast cereal—and vitamin D supplements.

And if you're prone to the winter blues, try to make the most out of what sunshine there is. Wrap up warm and enjoy a good walk—your vitamin D levels will thank you for it.

Want to try other foods for good moods? Cook up some cures after reading IDEA 21, *You are what you eat.*

Try another idea...

"*How heavy the days are. There is not a fire that can warm me, nor a sun to laugh with me.*"
HERMAN HESSE, *Steppenwolf*

Defining idea...

How did
it go?

Q   I've heard that taking a single but very high dose of vitamin D is as effective as light therapy. Would it do me any harm?

A   *It's important to remember that although vitamin D is a naturally occurring substance, it can be harmful. It is extremely toxic at high doses, so if you're tempted to crank up your dose, discuss it with your doctor first.*

Q   Is it really necessary to buy a light box? My husband is an artist and uses daylight effect lightbulbs. Could I sit by one of those?

A   *Sorry, but these lightbulbs just aren't up to the job. Light is measured in lux. The sort of full-spectrum bulbs used by artists that mimic natural light emit around 200–500 lux, whereas the lowest dose you can get away with to treat SAD is 2500 lux. Light boxes emit around 10,000 lux. Might sound high, but not when you realize the light emitted on a sunny day can be up to 100,000 lux. Which is a lot of lightbulbs.*

Q   I feel low every year when it starts to get dark earlier and have started using a light box every evening. I'm now having trouble sleeping. Could this be a side effect of light therapy?

A   *Sadly, yes. Light boxes can cause side effects. The most common ones are headaches, sore eyes, feeling squirmy, or problems getting to sleep. Try using your light box in the mornings instead and your sleep should improve.*

11
Nothing short of a miracle

Sometimes we all hope for miracles to get us through tough times. Ever considered conjuring your own? Discover a question that'll turn colossal problems into solutions of miraculous proportions.

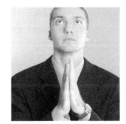

Ask a question, end up with a miracle.
I know, it sounds suspicious, but it's about finding what works and doing it often. Far easier than changing what you—or your friends and family—do wrong.

"Suppose one night there is a miracle while you are asleep and your problem is solved. What do you suppose you will notice different the next morning that will tell you there has been a miracle?" Insoo Kim Berg and Steve de Shazer are pros who figure it's easier to create solutions than solve problems. They ask their clients this question and it's part of what they call *brief solution-focused therapy*; it doesn't take long and it gets results. It's great for those of us wary of becoming therapy junkies. Don't get me wrong, some of my best friends are psychoanalysts, but if forty years of Freudian analysis hasn't flicked your switch, it's time to try this quirky quickie.

Here's an idea for you...

Be a time traveler for five minutes. Cast your mind back to the last thing you did really well. Perhaps it's bringing up four children on your own, rescuing your elderly neighbor from that ferocious toy poodle, or leaving your cheating boyfriend on the other side of the world before sneaking off and flying home with his return ticket and passport. Remind yourself how you did it. Where did you find your inspiration, muscle, or audacity?

It's easy to dismiss techniques that sound a bit too good to be true and that applies, oh, at least double when you're being offered a quick fix. So if you're thinking of skipping this chapter, stay right where you are. It might make you cringe but it can cure.

I suggest you grab a pen and paper, re-read the miracle question, and jot down imagined changes in as much detail as you can muster. Try to include small, telltale signs that would let you know there is something different. Who would be the first person to notice something different about you after the miracle? What would your partner/children/parents/friends/Pilates instructor notice was different about you if there had been a miracle? What would they all do differently? What would be different in your relationship with them?

Ronnie is a young widower who was depressed and lonely. Mornings were a nightmare of squabbling children who missed breakfast and were always late for school. He felt like a failure before the day had properly started. On a scale of 1 to 10, where 10 was the best Robbie had ever felt and 1 was suicidal despair, he gave himself a 3. Say Robbie woke up to find a miracle had happened. He'd bounce out of bed when the alarm rang instead of hitting the snooze button several times. The kids would get up without fighting with him or each other, and while they got ready, he'd make breakfast that they'd enjoy together before collecting packed lunches and heading off to school with plenty of time. People on his street, who had been avoiding him since his wife died five years ago, would respond to his smiles and newfound contentment. They would even notice how good looking he was. Robbie's life is pretty much like that now. He started doing some of the miracle solutions and now rates his mood as 8 out of 10. Want to try some of what he's got?

Finding it hard to imagine how life could be different? Check out IDEA 46, *Imagine*, to learn how to make your wildest dreams come true. (No, not the one about killing your boss.)

Try another idea...

Suspend reality and pretend your miracle has happened. And ask yourself these toughies: What will you need to do differently at work? What will you need to do differently at home? What will be the first thing your grumpy boss/bitchy colleagues/whining children will notice? What will they do differently?

If you've been jotting answers down, you might have had a Eureka moment. If you haven't, don't worry, it took me a while to get this, but to have the sort of changes in your life that it seems only a miracle could bring, you need to alter a few things. The catch? You're the one who does the altering. But you're already well on your way. Answering these questions helps you find ways out. So next time you think "only a miracle could get me out of this mess," remember: There can be a miracle, because you can produce one.

"I am realistic—I expect miracles."
WAYNE DYER, counselor who grew up in orphanages and foster homes

Defining idea...

How did it go?

Q   My problems are real. This miracle stuff seems a bit spurious. Are you seriously suggesting I pretend everything's fine and dandy?

A   *Sorry if I've been too flippant. I know your problems are real but, if you'll excuse me for sounding like an '80s televangelist, doing a few things differently can bring changes on a miraculous scale. If there are lots of things going on, I've found it helps to focus on the most urgent problem first. Give the miracle question a try and also ask yourself: How have I made things better in the past? How have I survived in spite of these problems? It might feel artificial because it's an unusual take on defeating depression but it really helps you discover success strategies and gets you to apply them to other problems.*

Q   I had a terrible childhood. Don't I need to understand and work through it before I can ever be happy?

A   *I can see why that seems logical, but there isn't a lot of proof that dissecting the past changes your future. In fact, dwelling on unhappy experiences may be stopping you from moving on. Imagine being lost on your way to a New Year's Eve party. Would you rather have a map showing the wrong turn you took three hours ago or directions to the party?*

12

All in the mind

Seeking respite from those dreary medical books simplified for (ahem) nonspecialist readers? This idea makes brain science shamelessly straightforward.

Ever wondered what's happening in your brain when you get depressed? And have you ever wondered how antidepressants change things? Time to take a trip inside the mind.

Too many depressed people are given brainless analogies. Maybe you've been told your batteries are flat and need recharging, or that your depression's like a broken leg that nobody else can see. Nonsense. Hippocrates, the father of medicine, taught his students that all suffering comes from the brain. This may not count as the latest finding from frontline research but he was right. When we're depressed, our brains work differently.

WHAT'S IN A BRAIN?

Your brain is a colony of ten billion interconnected cells that communicate with each other. Between each cell there are spaces called synapses. A synapse is a sort of junction between two brain cells, where the end of one almost touches another. Imagine you're talking to a friend and you're both on the bus. Easy, you just turn

53

Here's an idea for you... **Ask your physician or pharmacist to explain how your drugs work. A basic knowledge of brain chemistry will wow these pros and encourage them to explain correctly what's going on. There's no need to be condescended to with some cruddy explanation.**

and speak. But when you want to let your boyfriend know you'll be late because the bus is stuck in traffic, you use your phone. Cells use an equivalent of your mobile phone to communicate with each other across the synapse. Electrical charges are used to communicate inside brain cells. But electricity doesn't carry across the synapse, just as your voice doesn't carry outside the bus. So, while you'd use your phone, brain cells release chemical communicators. These chemical communicators are usually stored in little capsules called vesicles and when needed, swim into synapses, carrying their message to the next cell, ensuring communication carries on uninterrupted.

You've probably heard about these chemical communicators before. They're called neurotransmitters. Nobody knows for sure how many neurotransmitters there are, but at the last count there were over forty. They carry different messages. Some get their part of the brain turned on and excited, others put a damper on things. I promised not to blind you with science so I'll tell you about a couple of them and leave the other thirty-eight for a rainy day:

Serotonin drives our sleep and wake cycles. You might have heard that levels of serotonin are lower in people with depression. Instead of spreading communication in the synapse between adjacent brain cells, serotonin is reabsorbed, so communications about mood, sleep, appetite, and sex drive are lost.

Noradrenaline is like a party planner, controlling brain activity. But when you're depressed, noradrenaline is released from brain cells at a snail's pace, so activity levels plummet.

Learning about other ways of understanding depression can help you find new ways to make sense of low moods. Check out IDEA 25, *Schools of thought*.

Try another idea...

UNDER LOCK AND KEY

Brain cells are covered in receptors for these chemical communicators. In the same way that your house key only fits one front door on your street, receptors are shaped so that only one type of neurotransmitter will fit. Trying to get another neurotransmitter in the wrong receptor is just like the ugly stepsisters cramming their fat feet into Cinderella's glass slipper.

GREEN BRAINS

Your brain is a great recycler. Once neurotransmitters have done their thing, the brain cell that fired them out takes them back in. Pros call this reuptake. Many antidepressants work by stopping reuptake. Selective serotonin reuptake inhibitors (SSRIs),

"Men ought to know that from nothing else but the brain come joys, delights, laughter, grief, despondency, and lamentations."
HIPPOCRATES

Defining idea...

for example, prevent serotonin from being recycled, so there's more of it around, allowing those important brain signals to complete their journey.

How did it go?

Q **I've read about something called neurons and wondered if you can explain what they are?**

A   *Neuron is just a fancy word for brain cell.*

Q **If depression is just a chemical imbalance, why do so many people get better with talking treatments?**

A   *The jury's still out on this one. Some pros think our brain chemistry directly controls our emotions; others reckon our emotions directly control our brain chemistry. It's a bit of a theoretical debate though as either way, depression can spiral out of control if it's not treated with therapy or drugs.*

13

Go on, prove it

With a new miracle cure on every health page, how can you tell what works? Here's a guide to help you sort science fact from science fiction.

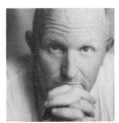

Sangam yoga, green tea enemas, or probiotic supplements may be the tabloid treatment of the week, but how do you know whether to hotfoot it to an alternative apothecary or give them the cold shoulder?

KEEP TAKING THE TABLOIDS

How do you know which claims to take at face value? Last week you read about a new drug for depression. Today you read it makes people aggressive and suicidal. It can be hard to know what to trust. There have always been quacks and charlatans tricking the vulnerable with "miracle" cures. But it's also true that many well-meaning people publish information on defeating depression that's confusing, unhelpful, or biased, so you need to be at least one step ahead of them. How? The short answer: by looking at scientific research. The long answer? Using key principles from evidence-based medicine. Confused? Hang in there, you soon won't be.

Buy a medical dictionary and a basic textbook and read up on the science behind the treatments you've been offered or are considering. The *Journal of the American Medical Association (JAMA)* **and** *Lancet* **are the most accessible medical journals for the layperson so are a good place to start. Many medical journals are now online, but it's well worth befriending a librarian first. She'll be able to show you how to search scientific literature online and how to access information.**

Evidence-based medicine. What is it? Evidence-based medicine, according to its originator, Professor Dave Sackett, is "conscientious, explicit and judicious use of current best evidence in making decisions about the care of individual patients."

JUST NOT HUMOROUS

Critics dismiss evidence-based medicine as a newfangled fad, but it dates back to the mid-nineteenth century. At that time, doctors still believed Hippocrates' physiological theory of the four humors. According to this theory, your health state of mind depended on a balance among the four elemental humors: blood, yellow bile, phlegm, and black bile.

In the 1830s, Parisian Pierre Louis challenged popular opinion of the efficacy of bloodletting. In a pioneering clinical trial, he kept meticulous records of treatments and outcomes of his patients, and was able to disprove the claims of the bloodletters. It was a bad time for French leech vendors.

DEVOUT SKEPTICS

Next time you hear or read about a new treatment, be skeptical and ask the following questions:

What's this claim based on? There's a pecking order for looking at research studies, as some are superior to others. The top two types of research papers are called meta-analyses and randomized controlled trials. In meta-analysis, researchers collect studies and comb through them. They trash any that don't meet strict criteria and combine results from the remaining high-quality research. Randomized controlled trials are studies that find out if a treatment works. People are split into groups but have an equal chance of ending up in either group. One group is known as the treatment group because they are given the new treatment. The other group gets an inactive treatment and is called the control group. Researchers then compare the effects of having the new treatment against having the inactive treatment.

If it is a randomized controlled trial, ask *Is this control group fair and relevant?* If one group has three green tea enemas a week, while the other group gets a five-minute phone call, the enema group might be getting better because they are having extra attention and human contact rather than green tea. On the other hand, if the control group has caffeine enemas and do get better, then there might be something in it.

Who paid for it? If research into sangam yoga is funded by the National Sangam Yoga Society, they've probably got a vested interest. You don't have to be a research expert to realize big bucks can cause preconceived notions or unfairly influence scientists or publishers.

Unhappy with your doctor's suggestion? Why not ask her what science says about your treatment? Find out how to work together, even when you disagree, in IDEA 38, *I did it my way.*

Try another idea...

"Show me the money!"
JERRY MAGUIRE

Defining idea...

How did it go?

Q **Do we really need all this scientific proof for everything when there are so many experts out there?**

A *Evidence-based medicine scientists think of expert opinion as the lowest form of medical evidence, even below flawed scientific research. Proponents of evidence-based medicine argue that opinion may be out of date, poorly recalled, or just plain wrong. The Center for Evidence-Based Medicine in Oxford, England, showed that textbooks don't mention many good treatments, even a decade after they've been shown to be effective. Even worse, libraries are stuffed with textbooks recommending treatments that have been shown to be useless. Opinion is based on, at best, a lifetime of clinical experience. Advocates of evidence prefer to base decisions on collective experiences of thousands of clinicians treating millions of patients, rather than depending on their own comparatively limited experience. A lot of popular opinion originates from drug companies. Call me cynical, but I reckon their user-friendly treatment guidelines are likely biased in favor of their company's product.*

Q **Aren't you potentially dismissing patients' perspectives on depression in favor of an average treatment effect?**

A *Good point. I accept it's not always straightforward deducing whether research evidence ought to be applied to a particular person. Research papers aren't able to tell you which treatment is ideal for you. Evidence-based medicine never set out to dismiss different perspectives, it just advocates integrating expertise with the best available research evidence.*

14

Diversion ahead

Problems, troubles, efforts, struggles. Life's rarely straightforward. But going over and over difficulties is guaranteed to make you feel even worse. Discover how to stop those melancholic musings.

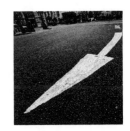

Same old thoughts going around in circles? Here's how going retro and revisiting your Rubik's cube can help.

RUINOUS RUMINATIONS

I don't need to tell you that when we're depressed, we spend hours mulling over problems and worries. Before you have a moment's peace to try to tackle 'em you're weighed down and distressed. Sound familiar? I call these spinning thoughts "ruinous ruminations." Diverting your mind from them, by using what the trade calls "distraction techniques," helps you cut down on time spent brooding and also lifts your mood. When I first heard about distraction techniques, I thought they were just a fancy way of shying away from real life. I was way off. It's a great technique. Diverting your mind from pessimistic ponderings gives you back the reins when emotions are running riot. And as you're in this for the long haul, you'll have more energy to take a positive look at problems and sort them out. You'll be able to replace those thoughts with positive, or at least constructive, ones. Next time you notice your thoughts spinning, try out one of these four diversions:

Here's an idea for you... **Poke around in the attic and dig out your Rubik's cube. Next time ruminations start, put all your mental energy into getting at least one side of the same color. With regular use, your ruinous ruminations could be a thing of the past, too.**

Alphabet zoo (T is for Tarantula): Go through the alphabet sequentially, naming an animal for each letter. If it's too easy, restrict yourself to a category like wild animals or exotic pets.

Objects of desire: Focus on an object of desire. I like to imagine a Chippendale (chair, not stripper). You can choose something you own, or something you don't have but lust after. Anything from a Lladro figurine to an antique chamberpot is fine. As you imagine your object, describe it to yourself in as much detail as you can. If you find this difficult, you might find these questions useful:

- What is it for?
- Where is it?
- What is it made of?
- What does it feel like?
- What color is it?
- Does it smell like anything?
- How tall is it?
- How much does it weigh?

Space sense: Using each sense in turn, describe the space you are in when ruminations bother you. Kirk uses this. He gets disturbing thoughts of throwing himself under a train whenever he travels by public transportation. Who doesn't? To distract himself he asks himself the following questions:

- What do the other passengers look like?
- What might they do for a living?
- What else can I see around me?
- What can I hear in the train?
- Can I hear different noises as we come to each station?
- What are my hands resting on?
- What does that feel like?
- Can I feel my clothes on my body?
- What are the textures like?
- Can I feel my contact lenses in my eyes?
- What can I smell?
- Can I taste anything?

You can adapt these questions to any setting.

Think of a number: While you're at it, think of two: a big number and a small one. Take the small number away from the bigger one. Now take the smaller number away from your answer. Keep going as far as you can, even when you're into negatives. And no, you're not allowed to use your fingers.

Exercise takes distraction one step further by giving you added mood-boosting benefits. Check out IDEA 40, *Pedal pushers*. If that's too energetic for you, how about cozying up with a book as discussed in IDEA 31, *A novel idea*.

Try another idea...

"A man's life is what his thoughts make of it."
MARCUS AURELIUS

Defining idea...

How did
it go?

Q **My partner, Jake, says that these distraction exercises are just a way of me avoiding painful stuff and if I don't face up to why I'm depressed, it won't go away. Is he right?**

A *Jake's partly right. They won't produce long-term changes, but because they whittle down depressive thoughts, they lift low mood and leave you able to look at painful stuff and problem-solve without getting worse.*

Q **I tried counting backward from 1,000 the last time I felt unhappy, but I just couldn't concentrate and ended up thinking about the mess my life is in. What should I do next time?**

A *Of course, it's hard to concentrate when your mind is troubled. I know this sounds harsh, but when you're upset, giving in to ruinous ruminations just makes things worse. How about picking a lower number, say 100, and counting back in multiples of six. Or you could distract yourself by doing something physical like doing dishes, raking leaves, or loading the washing machine.*

Q **I try to distract myself by imagining that I've won the lottery and how I'll spend my windfall, but I quickly end up thinking nothing first-rate like that would happen to me and it makes me more dejected about being in debt. Can you suggest anything?**

A *Fantasies can lift us out of humdrum daily grinds or they can have the opposite effect. In depression, positive thoughts are overpowered by negative ones so happy scripts we write in our mind are quickly spliced out or overwritten. The best distraction exercises use concentration but not imagination, so they shouldn't grind you down in the same way.*

15

Magnetic attraction

Can magnets max your mood? Magnets and the forces they produce can change the way you feel. Sounds wacky, I know, but transcranial magnetic therapy has a lot going for it.

Feeling repelled by the idea of a magnetic treatment for depression? Charlatans and swindlers have advertised suspicious magnetic cures for decades, but this reputable new technique is different.

Chinese medical practitioners have used magnetic treatments for depression for the last two millennia and some Tibetan monks alleviate depression using magnetic forces. As an up and coming junior psychiatrist (OK, I'd seen my first three patients with depression), I was asked to help with a trial investigating a pioneering treatment using magnets. I liked what I saw.

ELECTRIC DREAMS

Patients with severe, life-threatening depression are sometimes treated with electroconvulsive therapy (ECT). ECT is the most powerful antidepressant we've got,

Here's an idea for you... **You may be able to try transcranial magnetic therapy by taking part in a trial. Why not ask your doctor if this is being offered locally?** and unlike drugs, it works instantly, which can literally be lifesaving for people who are so depressed they have stopped eating and drinking. It has its fans, but also harsh critics. Many people who've had ECT have suffered from lasting memory problems so it's no longer used in several countries, including Holland. During ECT, electricity is fired through the brain, causing uncontrolled brain activity, resulting in a fit. TMS distributes it's get-up-and-go in a more controlled way. Unlike ECT, you don't need an anesthetic and it doesn't jumble your memory. Being awake means you can chat or read during treatment. This promising new treatment for severe depression is useful for depression that's stubbornly resistant to drugs.

WIRED UP

Here's how it works: Magnetic fields are produced by passing current through a handheld coil placed on your scalp to modify goings-on in your brain. TMS machines were developed twenty years ago as a tool to help scientists understand how the brain works without opening it up, which as you can imagine gets a little inconvenient. Placing magnets over a brain area involved in movement stimulated brain activity and triggered muscle twitches. For example, motor areas of your brain can be stimulated to make your thumb twitch, neatly demonstrating that nerve pathways are intact. Experts can use TMS to change movement, memory, reaction times, speech, and mood. This is how TMS can treat a number of illnesses, including depression.

IF THE CAP FITS...

During treatment, you wear a funky cloth hat that looks like a bathing cap, but with lines drawn on it so your doctor can see exactly where to place and hold the magnet. A powerful magnetic coil is then held over a place at the front of your head called the left dorsolateral prefrontal cortex—it's just behind your forehead. Big judgments, planning, and decisions get made there. There's strong evidence suggesting that the left prefrontal cortex is underactive in depression. Many people think TMS works by heightening this activity.

TMS is thought to work by inducing an electromagnetic current in certain brain cells. This affects neurotransmitter release. Confused? You won't be after IDEA 12, *All in the mind*, which makes brain science easy to come to grips with.

Try another idea...

POWERFUL PAINLESS PULSES

As the doctor holds the magnet, a number of painless magnetic pulses pass through your skull. This process makes a noise a little like a pecking woodpecker. These pulses induce electric currents, altering and aiding brain activity. Each treatment lasts around twenty minutes. Unfortunately, rather than just hooking up, getting zapped, and bouncing out, you need a course of treatment, usually every day or three times a week for two weeks.

"Stars open among the lilies.
Are you not blinded by such expressionless sirens?
This is the silence of astounded souls."
SYLVIA PLATH

Defining idea...

WHITE KNIGHT OR WHITE ELEPHANT?

We've been trying to find a good alternative to ECT for some time. Many people think TMS could be it, but others remain to be convinced. Preliminary results from trials on real people with real depression are promising, but it could still be some time before it's available at a clinic near you.

How did it go?

Q I've come across something called rTMS. What's that?

A When magnetic stimulation is pulsed at regular intervals, it is sometimes called repetitive TMS, which gets shortened to rTMS.

Q I've had electroconvulsive therapy three times and like the sound of TMS. Are there any side effects?

A ECT is used to treat severe depression. As you know, electrodes are put on your scalp to trigger electrical stimulation. But whereas TMS creates targeted activity, ECT creates widespread brain stimulation and so more side effects. Sadly, TMS isn't free of side effects. Headaches are common. TMS has caused epileptic fits in a few people.

Q How effective is TMS compared to other physical treatments?

A In various trials, TMS is usually found to be as helpful as antidepressant drugs, although the jury is still out as to whether it is as successful as ECT.

16

The CAT that gets the cream

Having another bad day? Wanna feel like the CAT that got the cream? You're just sixteen weeks from happiness with cognitive analytic therapy.

"Why do I always end up feeling like this?" You'll be able to answer this and other questions like it with this super chic but no-nonsense therapy.

Cognitive analytic therapy, CAT to you and me, was developed by Dr. Anthony Ryle, a psychiatrist at Guy's Hospital in London, as a way of treating people in a short time. Most people have sixteen sessions, but you may need as few as four. Ryle's research showed CAT is a safe and effective depression treatment.

WHAT'S IN A NAME?

Cognitive means using your views and thoughts about yourself.
Analytic means getting down to the nitty-gritty of the forces that drive what you do. Your relationship with the therapist is also thought to be important and used to help.
Therapy means helping you defeat depression through increased self-awareness. An aim of CAT is to give you tools for life.

Here's an idea for you...

Keep a diary of your mood and actions. It'll be a great help when you go for an assessment. If you keep a diary while waiting for therapy, you may get even more out of cognitive analytic therapy and it could shorten your treatment.

Many people feel stuck, powerless, and angry that unhelpful ways of thinking and doing things seem to happen over and over. In CAT, you'll work with a therapist and look at what has slowed down or stalled positive changes in your past. Unlike other talking treatments, CAT puts the spotlight on how problems develop and shows you what's wrong with your ways of coping with bad times.

But this isn't just a clever off-the-shelf package. The thing that makes this therapy a winner is that it's adapted to your life. By the end of the treatment, you'll understand how your unique coping techniques developed and how you can modify and improve them. Your strong points are the power for change. How marvelous is that? Extremely.

THE WAY I SEE IT

You'll be asked to tell your story and the therapist will start to understand more about your life and what makes you tick. When starting CAT, you'll be asked to fill in a questionnaire about common problems. CAT therapists often ask you to keep a record of your moods. After about four sessions, you'll be given something called a reformulation letter. This describes your life so far, difficulties you've struggled with, how you've survived them, and some new ways of seeing your problems. There'll usually be plenty of time for you to think about these observations and make factual changes. You'll either learn something about yourself you didn't know before, or see something you've never noticed before. Just one of these could open the door to lasting happiness. When you've both agreed on a way of setting out your difficulties and understanding them, you'll come up with some so-called *target problem procedures* and will work on them during the remaining sessions. People are often given a diagram showing how their past may be causing current problems. CAT therapists don't promise to cure you in sixteen weeks, but they'll give you the tools to finish the job.

If you've found the letter writing helpful, why not try keeping a diary? Discover how to write wrongs in IDEA 4, *Dear diary*.

Try another idea...

You'll need to do some homework between sessions, usually monitoring thoughts, actions, and feelings. These notes are used in CAT to give you a better understanding of how to make positive changes.

BREAKING UP IS HARD TO DO

Your last three sessions look at ending therapy and how this might affect you, especially if other endings or good-byes have been difficult. As well as talking about endings, you'll consolidate key themes from your work together. One of the things I really like about CAT is that you and the therapist exchange a "good-bye" letter, giving you both a chance to reflect and look back on the sessions. It's a tangible reminder of your own power to change.

Most therapists will offer a final appointment a couple of months after finishing therapy to see how things are going.

How did it go?

Q **I've had problems with depression for as long as I can remember and can't believe it could take just sixteen weeks to solve them. I like the sound of this approach, but wonder if it's ever offered for longer?**

A *Absolutely. Although unlimited or open-ended CAT is rare, having twenty-four sessions isn't at all unheard of. Sixteen weeks is a guide, but the actual length depends heavily on you and your therapist.*

Q **I seem to be able to find gurus, experts, and therapists working in every other style of therapy, but I'm unable to find anyone who offers CAT. Is there a central register?**

A *In a perfect world, there'd be a CAT therapist in every neighborhood, but there are lots of people in the same predicament as you. A good place to start is contacting your countries' association of cognitive analytic therapists. Ask them for a list of local therapists. It could be the start of a life-changing relationship.*

Q **I'm reluctant to go into therapy again since the last time I tried I became over-dependent on my therapist. This seemed to compound my problems. Will this happen with CAT?**

A *The beauty of CAT is that it is time limited. You know when the end will be from your first session and you and your therapist will be working on things you can do once sessions are over. The great thing about the final review appointment is that having said good-bye and exchanged good-bye letters, there is a safety net without the risk of dependence.*

17

On top of the world

High self-esteem makes you happier. Revving yours up should be a snap if you follow these simple rules.

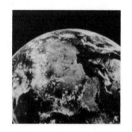

Want to be a happy, successful, sexy beast? Pull up a comfy chair and prepare to overhaul your outlook.

Self-esteem's a combination of how much you think you're worth and how accepted you feel. High self-esteem helps you cope with setbacks and makes you more immune to depression. Value yourself highly, and you'll also be more creative, resilient, and successful.

SPREAD YOUR ASSETS

You've probably noticed different parts of your life go well at different times. Work's going well, you're getting along with your partner, but all your kitchen appliances break down, one after another. Or you've fallen in love, but are out of a job with no sign of one on the horizon. No rhyme or reason to it, just life. The trouble is, if your self-esteem is all tied up with one part of your life, when that part goes badly, you're more at risk for depression.

73

Here's an idea for you...

Forget perfection. Try setting your goals below the superhuman threshold for a week and see your self-esteem soar. When we set our goals too high, we hardly ever reach them. When we do, it's amazing, but the rest of the time, we feel worthless and valueless.

Gerald, a real estate agent, gets depressed most winters. He thought it was seasonal affective disorder until he realized during a quiet year in the property market that his depression was closely connected with his work. When he got a lot of commissions, he felt on top of the world, but when sales were slow, Gerald felt like a failure. If you're getting all of your feel-good factor from one aspect of your life, it's time to spread your assets. Develop other areas like friendships, family ties, hobbies, and sports. That way, if you're laid off, your wife leaves you for an older man, and your roof falls in, your prize marigolds and pals from the Knights of Columbus might just see you through.

BE A BIG FISH IN A SMALL POND

What if you're on top of your game but not feeling on top of the world? Psychologist and writer Oliver James reckons high-flyers see themselves negatively because they compare themselves with other people in their league. This makes them lose sight of how well they're doing. "Their success leads to even further subordination," says Oliver, "because, having been one of the biggest fish in a pond, they are moved to a bigger one where they are just one in a shoal of equally high achievers." You don't need to ditch your business suit to bump up your self-esteem, but showing off in a beginners line dancing class, rather than making a fool of yourself in advanced footwork, is a good first step.

DITCH THE BITCH

Friends influence the way we see ourselves. A jealous girlfriend might persuade you your butt looks gigantic in those jeans, just because she can't afford them. Ditching friends who make you feel bad is one of the most effective self-esteem boosters going.

Are you always saying yes to placate friends and family? IDEA 29, *Just say no*, will help you become more assertive.

Try another idea...

Time for an address book audit. Look through your friends and ask yourself two serious questions:

■ Who helps me feel good about myself?
■ Who makes me feel small and insignificant?

Be ruthless. If someone cuts your confidence, slash them from your party list. Instead, spend your day off with people who boost your morale and encourage and support you.

SNUFF OUT THE ZAPPER

You know that little voice inside that whispers things like "You're a lousy mother," "Nobody wants to go out with you," and "You never do anything right"? He's the self-esteem zapper and it's time to do him in. Listen to the zapper and eventually you'll stop trying and give up. He sets you up to fail, stops you from noticing accomplishments, which he says are "just good luck," and is an all-around bad guy. Next time the zapper pipes up, think back over what happened and remind yourself of all the details. That should shut him up.

"The things we hate about ourselves aren't more real than things we like about ourselves."
ELLEN GOODMAN, journalist

Defining idea...

How did it go?

Q **I ditched all my critical friends but now I'm lonely. Help! What should I do?**

A *Friendships thrive on shared experiences. Evening classes, political groups, sports clubs, or volunteering can help you find people with similar interests. Once you've met people you'd like to spend more time with, keep in contact and develop your listening skills. Once you've shown you care, good friends will reciprocate.*

Q **I'm worried these tips will make me cocky and conceited. Isn't it selfish to put myself first?**

A *I used to worry about this and it almost got to the stage where I didn't do anything without thinking deeply about what effect it would have on everyone else. Trouble is, you can't please everyone all of the time. And living to please others leaves you feeling manipulated and exploited in the long run.*

Q **Most of my friends are supportive and kind. My problem is that I had a hypercritical dad who died ten years ago. He got into my head and I hear him berating my achievements and pouring cold water on any aspiration I have. How can I ditch him?**

A *Every time you hear his voice, use it as a cue to remind yourself he's gone and that his disapproval can't hurt or hinder anymore. Enlist the support of your helpful friends and lay him to rest once and for all. Is there a more positive father figure among them?*

18

Mind your mind-set

When you're depressed, certain mind-sets hamper your recovery and make misery more likely. Find out what you can do about it.

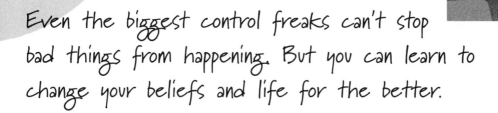

Even the biggest control freaks can't stop bad things from happening. But you can learn to change your beliefs and life for the better.

EASY AS ABC

Things that happen to us, how we experience these events, and how they make us feel are intimately interconnected.

- **A** is for **action**. Something happens. Maybe you don't land the dream job, your butt looks big in those jeans, your blind date stands you up, and everyone else gets invited to the party
- **B** is for **belief**. What do you believe about what happened? Belief is the spin we put on things. Any of these sound familiar? "Things always go badly for me," "I'm just a sad case," "That's so unfair," "Why me?," "That's just typical."
- **C** is for **consequences**. What if this belief is true? If I really believe I'm a sad case, how does that make me feel? How will it make me act? How will colleagues, friends, and family respond to me?

Here's an idea for you...

Undermine unhelpful mind-sets by acting against them. For instance, if you're working extra hard to prove your self-worth, give yourself a night off. If you're plagued by perfectionism, force yourself to accept less than 85 percent for a change.

MIND OUT

When you're depressed, certain entrenched mind-sets hamper your recovery and make depression more likely to come calling again. These five ways of thinking make people more prone to depression.

1. *Can't live without you (or without your approval).* I have to be a people pleaser all the time. If you don't love me, I'm nothing. As long as everyone likes me, I'm happy. I can't bear it if people are angry or criticize me. I need people to approve of what I'm doing.

2. *It's got to be perfect.* I must never make mistakes. I've got to look like a million dollars. I really ought to keep producing excellent results. If this book doesn't win the Nobel Prize, I've failed.

3. *I make the world go round.* Without me, everything falls apart. When things go wrong, it's usually my fault.

4. *Work to live.* As long as I'm working, I'm happy. I have to be prolific to be valuable.

5. *It's my right.* I should get what I want and need. It's my right. It's not as if I'm being unreasonable. And I want it yesterday.

DIG DEEP

Some of these mind-sets might be familiar, but you'll probably need to do a little detective work to see if there are any lurking behind more innocent-looking thoughts or assumptions. Using a technique called "the downward arrow" developed by Professor David Burns helps you identify unhelpful mind-sets, so you can work on them. Here's how it works. Next time something happens that makes you feel miserable or angry, write down what you're thinking. Draw an arrow under your thought and ask yourself "What if that was true? What would it mean?" Carolyn, a secretary, is feeling miserable and stressed. Here's how the downward arrow technique helps her see where these feelings come from:

If I don't type any faster, this letter won't be done in time for the lunchtime mail pickup.

What if this is true?
↓
What does it mean?

I'll miss my deadline and the letter won't get there by tomorrow.

What if this is true?
↓
What does it mean?

Not sure if your thoughts are really coming from an unhelpful mind-set? Experiment by putting your beliefs to the test in IDEA 35, *Doin' it differently*.

Try another idea...

"Most of the shadows of this life are caused by standing in one's own sunshine."
RALPH WALDO EMERSON

Defining idea...

79

Mr. Hunter will think I'm an awful secretary.

What if this is true?
↓
What does it mean?

He would think I was a failure.

What if this is true?
↓
What does it mean?

I'd feel very sad because I need his approval to feel happy.

What if this is true?
↓
What does it mean?

My happiness depends on people approving of what I'm doing.

Defining idea...

"I am an old man and have known a great many troubles, but most of them never happened."
MARK TWAIN

Once you've done the downward arrow several times, you'll probably identify some unhelpful mind-sets. There are things you can do to change them. Why bother? Remember the ABC? Change beliefs and consequences change, too. Like this:

- **List the pros and cons.** We cling to beliefs for reasons. It might seem crazy, but listing the pros and cons of your mind-set helps you see if there's anything in it for you.

- **Live with it.** None of us is perfect. Accepting yourself for what you are with thoughts like, "My butt does look big in this, but the rest of me looks OK" is more helpful than "Omigod, I'm a fat unlovable cow."

- **Peel off the label.** We tend to live up or down to labels, so calling yourself a loafer, no-hoper, degenerate, or other unpublishable name is a bad idea. Instead of saying, "I'm such a loser" try "I made a mistake. It happens to the best of us."

- **Call a friend.** Check out your thoughts with other people. Carolyn could ask her colleagues, "Do other people think I'm a bad secretary?"

- **Ditch the double standard.** I bet you're much harder on yourself than you are on your friends and family. Time to stop measuring yourself with a different ruler.

How did it go?

Q   **I'm an old, divorced, unemployed sad sack stuck in a studio apartment. How could your elaborate word games change that?**

A   *Regrettably, if you believe you're an old sad sack, you'll act like one and that's how others will treat you. Changing your beliefs can have a dramatic effect. Perhaps it's not your circumstances getting you down, but your view of them? Thinking of yourself as a footloose, fancy-free bachelor looking for the right opportunity is more likely to bring work and a little love to your life.*

Q   **I'm a perfectionist but can't see why it's a problem. Doesn't this just mean I'm a high achiever?**

A   *Maybe. All high flying go-getters want to get the job done and settle for less than 100 percent to meet deadlines. True perfectionists, on the other hand, aim to get things perfect, rather than get them done. If you'd rather not do something at all if you can't do it perfectly, I'll leave you to decide which camp you're in.*

19

I don't know what to do

Are you looking for ways of coping with problems that trigger depression? Try these tried and trusted problem-solving strategies.

Problems with partners, friends, health, work, or money often trigger depression. So it's hardly surprising that researchers at Oxford University found that problem-solving reduces depression, anxiety, and hopelessness.

Ready to get your hands dirty? Great. Follow this seven-step formula for problem-solving:

1. *Start by writing down problems that are contributing to your depression.* Melika did this and her list was as follows:
   - Having lots of arguments with Dad
   - Struggling to keep up car payments
   - Feeling lonely and cut off from people
   - Can't get a job
   - Nothing to wear

Here's an idea for you...

Instead of ruminating endlessly about all your problems to your friends, pick one or two critical issues and ask a friend to help you brainstorm solutions. Bouncing ideas off each other will help you come up with a richer list.

2. *Overwhelmed with problems? Pick one at a time.* No one can solve all her problems in one try. So choose the problem that worries you most or the one that just can't wait and put a star by it. Melika starred her last item, "nothing to wear," which surprised me, but she said it was stressing her out because she'd been invited to a party.

3. *Go from the general to the specific.* Once you've picked your problem, try to rewrite it in a specific way. Melika changed "nothing to wear" to "I can't decide whether to wear my little black Versace number or long red Moschino skirt." The reason it helps to be specific is that you'll know when your problem is solved. Once Melika decides what to wear, her most urgent problem is solved.

4. *Identify different options by brainstorming.* I know it sounds like a gimmick for advertising moguls, but it works.

    Now it's time to get out the flip-chart, or at least a big piece of paper. Scribble down as many possible solutions as you can. These questions should help:

    ■ What's worked before?
    ■ If my best friend had this problem, what would I suggest?
    ■ What would Mom, Dad, or Harry from the corner store advise?

    Include everything—even zany or outlandish stuff can help you think quickly and creatively.

    Jenna was depressed after months of bullying by her boss. Here are her brainstorm options:

    ■ Stab boss with letter opener
    ■ Confront him

- Stay out of his way
- Tell his boss

5. *Examine every solution, weighing pros and cons.* When you've got a list of options, think through the pros and cons of each. You might want to draw up a table.

Feeling too sluggish to brainstorm? Try IDEA 22, *Actions speak louder than words*, or IDEA 6, *A pleasure a day keeps the blues at bay*, to lift your mood first. You can always come back once you're more motivated.

Try another idea...

Jenna weighed her options like this:

Option	Pros	Cons
Stab boss with letter opener	It would get him off my case. He'd know what it feels like to be picked on. I'd feel better.	It's wrong. I'd get arrested and sent to prison. I don't really think I could do it. My friends would be disappointed in me.
Confront him	He would know that I see his behavior as bullying.	He might deny it or treat me even worse. Might be humiliating.
Stay out of his way	I wouldn't have to confront him.	Even if I ignore him, he'll still be there and will bully me. I'll have to do something about it eventually.
Tell his boss	I would feel better. Something might be done about his bullying.	I'm scared of telling on him. I don't know who his boss is. They might not believe me.

6. *Pick the solution that has the most pros.* As you think of the pros and cons, run each option through this two-question filter:

- Will it help?
- Can I do it?

"A problem well-stated is a problem half-solved."
CHARLES FRANKLIN KETTERING, inventor

Defining idea...

7. *Plan steps you'll take to put your chosen solution into action and go for it.* So what happened with Jenna? She confronted her boss. He denied everything so she went for her second option, speaking to his superior. It turns out he'd bullied before, so he was given his marching orders. She's much happier now.

How did it go?

Q   I can't see how making a list of my problems will make them go away. How can it?

A   *You're right. It won't. But problems have a knack for spiraling out of control and making a list is a first step to getting some control back. When we feel we've lost control, stress levels soar and depression runs riot. This strategy not only gives you control but helps you find solutions that work.*

Q   I'm in debt—how can I begin brainstorming ways out?

A   *Like many problems, debt is far too big to tackle in one shot. Perhaps you could break it up, a little like this:*

- *I can't keep up with payments on the house since interest rates went up.*
- *I've got store card bills rivaling third-world debt.*
- *It's my wife's fiftieth next week and I can't afford the eternity ring she's hinted about.*

Now choose the most pressing—probably keeping the roof over your head— and brainstorm. Your ideas will work best, but here are a few suggestions to help you generate creative ideas: shop around for a different mortgage; rent out your home to cover bills and move in with your in-laws; get a better-paying job; move to a smaller house. Once you've finished brainstorming, think your choices through and reject those that won't work for you. Run with one that does. Good luck.

20

Don't jump

When depression hits hard, life rarely feels worth living. Thought about ending it all? Read on for everything you ever needed to know about surviving suicidal feelings.

Many depressed people go through times when they feel there's no point carrying on—days, weeks, or even months when life's too much of a struggle.

If you've thought about hurting yourself, or ending your life, it doesn't mean you're crazy or past a point of no return. I know it's easy for me to say, but you can get through this. Many people who have felt as bad as you have recovered. If you're suicidal, ask yourself honestly if you want to die, or to feel better. Attempting suicide has never cured anyone of depression, but whatever is making you feel awful will pass and you'll be free from pain. The catch? You have to be alive to experience freedom.

When you feel suicidal, what holds you back? Who or what prevents you from putting your plans into action? List your deterrents and remind yourself of them when you feel like throwing in the towel. As well as more obvious stuff like

Here's an idea for you... **Knowing exactly where to find help could save your life. Invest five minutes in making a crisis card: a small card of emergency contact details you carry in your wallet. Look up the numbers of your doctor, any pros you're seeing, and the local emergency department. Record them all on one little index card. Done.**

religious beliefs, think about what you'll miss. Consider what you'd like to do once you recover. Maybe you've never been abroad or would miss seeing your daughter get married or your grandchildren grow up.

SUICIDE IS UGLY

When I was a teenager, I had a fairly romantic view of suicide. Hollywood has a lot to answer for: The jilted bride swallows a handful of pills and her handsome lover sweeps in with flowers and regrets. Real life couldn't be further from this sugary fantasy. As a doctor, I've seen many suicide attempts involving hefty doses of humiliation, shame, and discomfort. It's heartbreaking seeing people with organ damage or who are wheelchair-bound after inflicting lasting disability.

HELP, I NEED SOMEBODY

If you feel like acting on suicidal thoughts, get help fast. Talking about how you ended up feeling so distressed usually helps get back some stability. Is there someone you can call? Bear in mind family and friends might freak out about suicidal feelings. Try not to be too hard on them. Chances are they're scared and maybe feel upset or guilty for not taking better care of you. In these circumstances, some people find speaking to a stranger useful. If so, call a suicide-prevention hotline. Other people say speaking to someone who knows them helps. If this rings true, call your doctor and ask for an urgent appointment on the same day. Already in touch with a pro? Contact them for emergency help. Alternatively, go to your nearest emergency room and ask to speak to a psychiatrist.

Some people cope with distressing feelings by hurting themselves. Sound familiar? IDEA 37, *Cut it out*, gives you safe alternatives.

Try another idea...

GIVE YOURSELF A BREAK

Reminding yourself that suicidal feelings are temporary and part of depression can help you see other ways out. Even if suicidal feelings swamp you, it doesn't mean you have to end it. Tell yourself feelings aren't the same as actions. Even if you feel like killing yourself right now, it doesn't follow that you have to act right away. Make a pact not to act on self-destructive feelings for at least twenty-four hours. You have already done it for ten minutes, just by reading this idea. You can do it for another ten minutes by reading another. You'll discover even though you still feel suicidal, you're not acting on it.

"Any day is a good day to die, but no day is a good day to take your life."
JASON, teenager from New Mexico who survived a suicide attempt

Defining idea...

How did it go?

Q **I feel very down and don't want to be a burden on my family. I really do believe we'd all be better off if I was dead. How can that be selfish?**

A *I'm sorry you feel so unhappy. Many severely depressed people feel they're a burden on friends and family and, like you, believe that other people would be better off without them. Ten years ago, I felt like this, but it's important to understand this is your depression talking. Many people who recover from depression are relieved they didn't kill themselves. Two of my friends committed suicide and through my job I've seen the trail of devastation suicide leaves behind. Many families never recover. I don't think there's ever a time when families or friends are really better off facing a tragic, premature death.*

Q **My dad tried to kill himself by taking an aspirin overdose. Mom died two years ago and he misses her. He didn't do himself any harm, but I'm worried about him. My brother thinks he's frightened himself out of doing anything like that again. How can we be sure?**

A *You can't. I'm afraid your brother's not quite right about people scaring themselves. In fact, the opposite's true. Once someone has crossed that line, it becomes easier to cross it in the future. One in a hundred people who survive an overdose commit suicide the following year. Speak to your dad about what happened. It might feel awkward for both of you, but you'll get a better idea of what he's going through and how you can help. If he's actively suicidal or making plans to kill himself, don't hesitate to call in experts.*

21

You are what you eat

Sometimes we all feel only a jumbo-size chocolate bar or bag of chips can make us feel better. But comfort eating doesn't have to mean binges and elasticized waistbands. Learn how to exploit the relationship between your diet and depression.

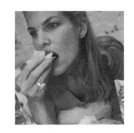

Bodies need many nutrients to generate the brain chemicals that influence our feelings. Want a diet to max your mood? Include these essential nutrients but go easy on unhealthy foods.

SWEET NOTHINGS

You don't need a book like this to tell you that when you eat something sweet, you get a head rush. But have you noticed, about an hour after that fifth doughnut, feeling as if you're going to pop, then feeling sleepy and perhaps even a teensy bit irritable? Why? When our moods dip, many of us reach for sugary foods or so-called "refined carbohydrates" like white bread, white rice, and processed foods. You're not going to like it but time-honored comfort foods give you mood swings. Another problem with these products is that they perpetuate craving cycles. When blood

Here's an idea for you...

Change your fattitude. Next time the urge to snack assails you, bypass the cookie jar and try one of these instead: rice cakes and cream cheese, a small handful of mixed nuts and fruit, banana and soymilk smoothie, low-fat cheddar cubes and apple slices.

...and another idea

Combine some mood-enhancing foods and create a delicious gourmet treat, like whole meal pasta with tuna, cheese, and pine nuts, to make your mouth water and mood soar.

sugar levels fluctuate wildly, this overstimulates glands, messing up your hormones and worsening depression. No prizes for realizing being overweight won't do much for your self-esteem either. Craving balance? Eating small, evenly spaced meals keeps your blood sugar levels and your mood steady.

TAKING A TRYP

Tryptophan, a building block of many proteins, has been used to treat depression successfully. Not so surprising if you know your brain has many naturally occurring chemical communicators. One of them is serotonin. When we're depressed, we have lower serotonin levels. Tryptophan is converted into serotonin in our bodies. Foods rich in tryptophan include: turkey, chicken, fish, pheasant, partridge, cottage cheese, bananas, eggs, nuts, wheat germ, avocados, milk, beans, peas, legumes, soy milk, pumpkin seeds, tofu, and almonds. Unfortunately, as tryptophan is just one building block and because it's fairly big, others that are more easily absorbed by your body will be taken up instead. The way around this is to divert the competition by eating starchy foods, like brown rice, whole meal bread, oats, and baked potatoes in the same meal as tryptophan-rich food.

OMEGA-3

Depression is about ten times more common in Europe and North America than in Taiwan. In fact, depression is pretty rare in places like Hong Kong and Japan where they eat a lot of fish. Scientists thought this might be because depression is related to omega-3 fatty acids, which are found in fish oils. Researchers investigating omega-3 supplements have found it helps severely depressed, even suicidal patients. Fish and seafood provide the complex omega-3 most important to the brain.

Don't eat fish? I'm afraid you'll need to count on your body converting a simpler fat called alpha-linolenic acid (ALA), into omega-3. The easiest way to include ALA in your diet is by munching nuts and seeds. Walnuts, brazil nuts, and flaxseed are your best bet. And go organic. Organic milk contains 70 percent more omega-3 than standard milk.

IRON MAN

If you're low in iron, you'll be tired and less likely to be up for any mood-boosting exercise. Rev up your iron stores by putting some red meat on the table at least twice a week. Roast beef, venison, and liver are all good sources.

Tryptophan helps in depression since it's one of the building blocks of serotonin. Want to learn more about brain chemistry? Check out IDEA 12, _All in the mind._

Try another idea...

"Let food be your medicine and your medicine be your food."
HIPPOCRATES

Defining idea...

How did it go?

Q **My teenage daughter is a strict vegan. Her father and I are worried this may be contributing to her depression. Could it be?**

A *Vegan diets can be very healthy, but the key here is balance. Get her to keep a diary of what she eats over a couple of weeks and run it by a dietician to check that she's getting enough calories and iron. Low levels of iron will make her feel tired and sluggish, which could pull her mood down.*

Q **I've heard chocolate is an antidepressant. How much do I need to take?**

A *This is a rumor, and one I often wish was true. Chocolate does contain a bit of tryptophan, but there are much richer sources. You're probably getting a rush from sugar and caffeine in chocolate but this is short-lived. Long term, lots of sugar and caffeine makes us feel worse. So, no prescriptions for a king-size chocolate bar. Life's unfair, isn't it?*

Q **When I see lists of food that are supposed to be good for you and others that are bad, I could weep. Everything, and I mean everything, I like is on the wrong list. What can I do?**

A *Yes, life is cruel. Over time your palate will adjust, and I know that because I've been there. I gravitate toward chocolate rather than celery, too, and I think most people do. The trick is to make it fun. Try including one new food item in your weekly shopping or make home-cooking look like junk food but with healthier ingredients.*

22

Actions speak louder than words

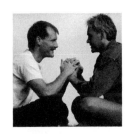

Spending too much time thinking that you're a pathetic loser and there's no point in doing anything? Find out why it's not what you do, it's the way you do it.

When you're depressed, it can be difficult to do all those things you usually do on autopilot. Small things like taking a shower and preparing a meal become marathon tasks.

THE DEPRESSIVE–SLUGGISHNESS CYCLE

Most people with depression do less than usual, and when we do less, we spend more time ruminating about troubles and uncertainties. And if that's not bad enough, the less you do, the less there is to get enjoyment from. After a short while, this makes you more depressed. Any residual motivation plummets. It's a cruel and vicious cycle sucking you deeper into despair and hopelessness.

Here's an idea for you...

List the activities that make you feel better. When you draw up next week's timetable, include as many of these activities as you can to max your odds of feeling better fast.

TURNING THE TABLES

One of the best ways of getting active again is by scheduling activities. Timetables help in two ways: Doing activities you enjoy or that give you a sense of accomplishment helps to reduce despair and hopelessness. Timetables can also expose relationships between activities and mood. For example, Fred noticed that playing tennis and cooking alone lifted his mood while having staying in bed and eating out had the opposite effect. You'll need to draw up a daily timetable, divided into one-hour slots from waking to bedtime. Fill in everyday jobs, household tasks, errands, odd jobs, any special responsibilities, and some entertaining activities. Although the idea of timetables might induce flashbacks of math class on Monday mornings, you'll honestly find it's easier to get going when you have a chart of what to do and when to do it. The first time I did this, I failed miserably, as all the tasks I set myself to do in an hour all took about three weeks. Avoid my blunder (and tears of frustration) by setting yourself small, achievable tasks first—writing a thank-you card to a friend rather than writing the next *Lord of the Rings*–type trilogy.

Defining idea...

"Iron rusts from disuse, stagnant water loses its purity, and in cold weather becomes frozen, even so does inaction sap the vigor of the mind."
LEONARDO DA VINCI

This idea works best when you include activities you enjoy, but you don't need a book like this to tell you that when you're badly depressed, nothing's fun anymore. The solution? Think back to the sorts of things that once gave you a buzz and include as many of them as you can. You could also include things you think you'd enjoy if you weren't depressed. Is there something you've always wanted to try? Put it on your list.

AT THIS RATE...

As you complete each routine or fun activity, rate each one for the amount of enjoyment and accomplishment you get out of it, on a scale of 1 to 10, where 10 is the highest. As days turn to weeks, then months, you'll see activities getting easier and recognize achievements that depression often blinds us to.

IDEA 7, *The time of your life*, **shows you how to boost your chances of accomplishing daunting tasks by tackling them in manageable pieces.**

Try another idea...

To help you get the idea, here's one I made earlier:

Time	Task	Enjoyment	Accomplishment
7 a.m.	Get out of bed	2	7
8 a.m.	Wash and dress	5	7
9 a.m.	Make and eat breakfast	4	6
10 a.m.	Listen to radio	6	5
11 a.m.	Go out for walk	7	4
12 noon	Read newspaper	6	8
1 p.m.	Make and eat lunch	4	5
2 p.m.	Laundry	5	7
3 p.m.	Buy meal for later	7	6
4 p.m.	Listen to music	8	5
5 p.m.	Put away laundry	5	7
6 p.m.	Candlelit bath	8	7
7 p.m.	Eat prepared meal	8	2
8 p.m.	Call John	7	7
9 p.m.	Check email	6	8
10 p.m.	Get ready for bed	5	5
11 p.m.	Read in bed	7	6

How did it go?

Q   **Oh, dear. I can't even find the energy to plan my week. What do you suggest?**

A   *Consider breaking this task down into manageable chunks. Start by making a list of chores and essentials like eating and brushing your teeth. When you've finished, make a second list of fun stuff. Find a friend to help you put the essentials into a timetable and include something to look forward to every day.*

Q   **I've been doing this for a few weeks and although I've noticed my enjoyment scores improving, I don't seem to accomplish much. My highest accomplishment score is still only 3. Why?**

A   *Stress not, this happens to lots of people. When we're depressed, we underestimate success. My guess is you're concentrating exclusively on what you haven't done, rather than noticing what you've attained. Dwelling on how much easier things were before you became depressed? Try to make allowances for how depression makes it difficult to do things.*

Q   **I've tried these timetables but they haven't worked for me. My enjoyment score is only 2 or 3. How can I do better?**

A   *In my book, anything's better than 0/10. Doing something is always better than doing nothing: 2 or 3 might not seem like much now but it's a start and something you can build on. Take comfort in what you've managed to score so far. This'll give you the impetus to keep going and, in time, enjoy life even more.*

23

Don't panic

Have you suddenly become afraid of the dark? Depression and anxiety go hand in hand. Try these strategies for managing panic attacks, free-floating anxiety, and all those irrational fears.

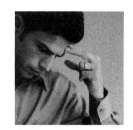

Feeling stressed and anxious? It's hardly surprising. Depression's hard to cope with and it means the small stuff is more likely to get you down.

SABER-TOOTHED TIGERS

Anxiety is caused when your primeval fight or flight mechanism gets activated. This device evolved as a survival strategy when confronted by, say, a saber-toothed tiger. It kicks in when you feel under threat. At low levels, increased anxiety leads to better performances. Low-level stress is essential for survival, enabling you to produce work to high standards. But adding extra stress when you've already reached your peak can have catastrophic results. Typically, tiredness is the first sign. Exhaustion and illness follow if stress continues unchecked.

Here's an idea for you... **Visit a self-help or support group and discover how other people have overcome anxiety. You may find other people have developed techniques that work well for you.**

PANIC ATTACKS

Ever felt suddenly and overwhelmingly afraid? Maybe thinking you were going to go crazy or die? If you had some of these symptoms, it was a panic attack:

- Racing or pounding heartbeat
- Chest pain
- Dizziness
- Difficulty breathing
- Tingling hands
- Feeling disconnected from everything or everyone
- A feeling that something unimaginably horrifying is about to happen
- Fear of going crazy
- Fear of dying

Panic attacks last about ten minutes, but when you're having one it can feel a lot longer. They're one of the most frightening and upsetting things you can go through.

What can you do about them? The first thing to remember is that all of these strange symptoms are completely harmless. They can't make you have a heart attack or stroke, and you're not going crazy. They all happen because your body has had a sort of false alarm, kicking you into saber-toothed tiger fighting mode. Panic attacks are a case of right feelings, wrong place, wrong time. Breathing deeply and slowly counteracts the effects of this fight or flight reaction.

Panic attacks feel awful because you misinterpret the signals your body is giving you. Tell yourself those palpitations and rapid, shallow breaths are just your body's way of preparing you to fight the tiger. Many people fear they'll faint, making a fool of themselves. Sound familiar? Next time remind yourself that when the fight or flight response kicks in, your blood pressure rises, making fainting physiologically impossible.

A massage is a great way to calm down. No personal masseuse? Now you don't need one because IDEA 43, *All hands on deck*, shows you how to give yourself a head massage to DIY for.

Try another idea...

ANXIETIES AND PHOBIAS

Many people with depression are also in a state of near-constant worry. You might feel tense, sweaty, or sick. Many people feel jumpy and on edge or find it hard to swallow.

Phobia means irrational fear. Sufferers know things like the dark, dogs, or elevators can't harm them, but feel irrationally scared and avoid them if they can.

CBT

Cognitive behavior therapy, that's CBT to you and me, can help you cope with anxiety-provoking situations, often by exposing you to them. It might seem counterintuitive but it helps to tackle the symptoms. CBT shows you that many terrifying thoughts are harmless. As you learn to no longer fear the sensations and scary thoughts, you become less and less afraid of panic.

"Anxiety is a thin stream of fear trickling through the mind. If encouraged, it cuts a channel into which all other thoughts are drained."
ARTHUR SOMERS ROCHE, writer

Defining idea...

101

SELF-HELP

Make a list of all the feelings you have during a panic attack and what you think they mean. Next, do some research into anxiety and find out what's really going on. Make a list or table and keep it in your bag or pocket. List "Feelings," "What I think this means," and (from your research) "What else could it mean?" For example: *Feeling*, "I've got pins and needles in my hands and the tips of my fingers are going numb"; *What I think this means*, "I'm going to have a stroke and will probably die"; *What else could it mean?*, "This numbness is a symptom of hyperventilation. If I slow down my breathing it will get better. It won't harm me." Next time you feel anxious, get the list out to remind yourself of what's really going on.

Q **When I have a panic attack, I'm sure I'm going crazy. How can I be sure that I'm not?**

How did it go?

A *Millions of people around the world have panic attacks every day and, like you, many of them think they are going crazy. In my book, going crazy means becoming psychotic or losing touch with reality. As far as I know, nobody has ever become psychotic by having a panic attack. I reckon you're more likely to win the lottery ten weeks running than be the first.*

Q **Can CBT techniques help with depression as well?**

A *Absolutely. There's a mass of evidence that CBT is as effective as antidepressants in mild to moderate depression.*

Q **I've heard that medication called benzos can stop panic attacks. Do you think they could help me?**

A *Please don't go there. Benzodiazepines, to give them their full name, were better known in the past as "mother's little helpers." Using them to treat panic attacks is a major no-no because they are horribly addictive and cause so-called rebound anxiety, meaning all your symptoms come back with a vengeance when you try to come off them. Some antidepressants are good for panic attacks and are not addictive, so why not ask your doctor about them? In the meantime, I suggest you check out some self-help techniques and see a good CBT therapist.*

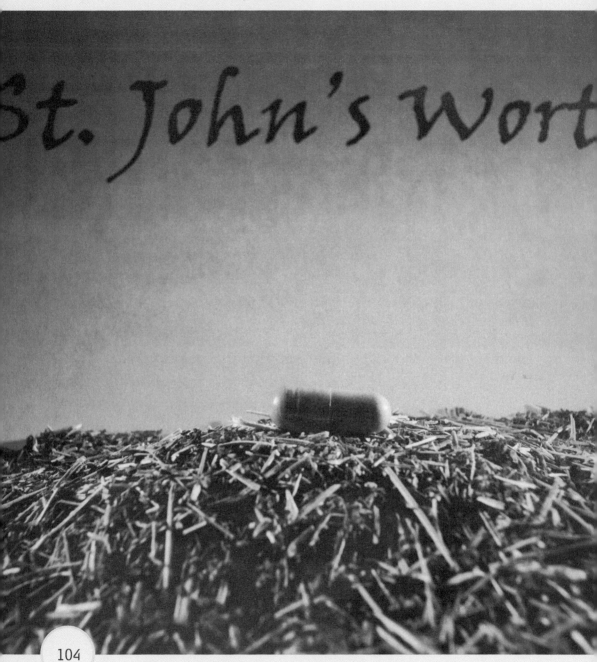

24

Natural highs

Poised to pop an herbal helper? What makes an herb nature's Prozac rather than a noxious plant? This idea may be hard to swallow but it might just save your life.

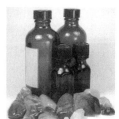

Lavender, borage, and ginkgo biloba have been plugged as herbal cures for depression. Some so-called natural remedies deliver everything they promise on the label. Others are ineffective impostors or even a toxic rip-off.

WORTS AND ALL

Good scientific evidence that herbal treatment works is pretty scant. So it was a welcome surprise when a little yellow shrub named after a saint caused a stir in the *British Medical Journal*. Researchers showed it to be effective in treating people with mild or moderate depression.

What was the magic weed? *Hypericum perforatum*. Sounds like a Harry Potter spell, so most of us call it by its other name: St. John's Wort. It grows in many parts of the world including Europe and the United States, and has been used as an herbal remedy for around two thousand years. In Germany, it tops the antidepressant bestseller list, outselling Prozac 20 to 1. It's available as a dried herb, liquid, tincture, and tablet.

Here's an idea for you...

Talk through the pros and cons of taking St. John's Wort with your doctor. If you decide to go for it, you'll need to take it for at least four weeks before it starts to lift your mood.

Getting ahold of St. John's Wort can be difficult; I'm afraid it depends where you live. In some countries, like Germany, St. John's Wort is a licensed medication and hundreds of thousands of prescriptions get written every year. In other places, like the UK, it isn't licensed so can't be prescribed. Although you might be able to buy St. John's Wort without a prescription in health food shops or pharmacies, depression is a serious illness and it's never a good idea to self-medicate.

You need to take 900 mg of the active ingredient hypericin every day for it to be effective. Unfortunately, many brands contain much less, so it pays to check the small print. Hypericin works on brain chemistry like conventional antidepressants. When you're depressed, there's an imbalance of a brain chemical called serotonin. Hypericin corrects this imbalance by recycling it. You should start to feel better after about six weeks.

NO SIDESTEPPING

Defining idea...

"If nature can offer us sound, safe, legal antidotes to the poisoning of the human spirit, then there can be no more important work in the twenty-first century than researching and exploring these resources."
STING

Rigorous scientific trials mean there's a lot to be said for conventional medicine. But, if you've ever taken them, you'll know conventional antidepressants cause a lot of side effects including headaches, nausea, sexual dysfunction, insomnia, heart rate abnormalities, weight changes, short-term memory loss, and rashes. No big surprise that they don't suit everyone. The good news is that St. John's Wort has fewer side effects than non-herbal antidepressants. Sadly, this doesn't mean there aren't any. Some people find their skin burns more easily in the sun. If you're taking St. John's Wort, you might feel sick, tired, or form a deep and meaningful relationship with your lavatory.

If you want to learn more about how to separate science fact from science fiction, check out IDEA 13, *Go on, prove it.*

Try another idea...

HARD TO SWALLOW

St. John's Wort also plays dirty tricks on your liver. It interacts with something called the cytochrome P450 enzymes. If, like me, you haven't got a degree in molecular hepato-chemistry, this means half a pharmacist's stock won't work properly if you take them with St. John's Wort. Might not sound like a big deal, but look over the list below and you'll see that combining like a herbal happy pill with something you've been taking for years can have calamitous consequences, from unplanned pregnancies to rejected kidney transplants or even death. Scary.

So don't take St. John's Wort if you're already taking any of these:

- Contraceptive pill
- Certain migraine, cancer, hypertension, epilepsy, asthma, and HIV drugs (check with your doctor)
- A selective serotonin reuptake inhibitor
- Warfarin
- Digoxin
- Cyclosporin
- Statins and other cholesterol-lowering drugs
- Carbamazepine

"The cheering effects of herbs and alliums cannot be too often reiterated."
PATIENCE GRAY, food author

Defining idea...

107

How did it go?

Q **You say that St. John's Wort is suitable for mild or moderate depression. I feel dreadfully depressed. What does mild or moderate mean?**

A *Good question. Depression is a complex continuum with normal sadness at one end and serious illness at the other. In the trade we assign people to one of three arbitrary points: mild, moderate, and severe. Most people are at the mild to moderate end. Deciding how severe an episode is depends on the number and intensity of certain symptoms, including sleep disturbance, appetite and weight change, anxiety, poor concentration, irritability, and suicidal thoughts. To find out how severe you own depression is, get diagnosed by a pro.*

Q **My mother-in-law takes ginseng and swears by it. Are the other herbs you mention no good?**

A *I know this sounds stuffy, but there just isn't enough scientific evidence to be sure ginseng or other herbs are useful antidepressants. Manufacturers make lots of bold claims and many herbs have a loyal fan base. I wouldn't take a biologically active substance that may scramble my brain chemistry without research showing it was at least as effective as the best of what we've already got. Not convinced? Many people took the herbal extract ma huang, claiming it gave them more energy. It's now been banned in the United States after being linked to 155 deaths. But hold the hate mail. I'm not saying all alternative therapy is claptrap. Just beware of holdover hippies selling hemp cures.*

25

Schools of thought

All those professionals can be really confusing, with everyone saying different and seemingly contradictory things. Finding out what's really what lets you take your pick.

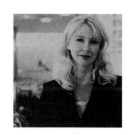

What makes you depressed? With dozens of different theories, from imbalanced brain chemistry to disrupted childhoods, it's time to take stock. Mine this wide range of approaches to create explanations that make sense to you.

Different professional training leads to various ways of assessing, explaining, and treating depression. Although it can be irritating and confusing, there are various ways of understanding and explaining depression. Rather than sticking your head in the sand, finding out about different schools of thought helps you understand depression and make informed choices about therapies and treatments.

DISEASE MODEL

This one you probably know about. Many professionals explain depression in terms of physical pathology. Brain chemicals, known as neurotransmitters, affect our moods.

Here's an idea for you... **List the factors that might make you more prone to depression—it's unlikely there's one single cause. Then consider what could have triggered this particular episode—your family history or a key life event, for example. Finally, ask yourself what's stopping you from getting better. Thinking through this rubric using different schools of thought will give you new ideas for defeating depression and can focus your attention on areas you hadn't considered important.**

Low levels of the neurotransmitter serotonin lead to depression. Receive the right antidepressant and your symptoms will subside.

BEHAVIORAL MODEL

Behaviorists introduced the behavioral model. Burrhus Frederic Skinner believed behaviors that aren't reinforced by food, money, or social attention fade away. He thought behavioral patterns in depression were due to the absence of reinforcement.

Martin Seligman developed a theory of depression that he called the "learned helplessness theory." He demonstrated this on dogs. Seligman's dogs were repeatedly presented with a warning signal followed by an electric shock. At first, the dogs tried to escape when they heard the signal, but when they couldn't they gave up. Later, he gave the dogs an escape route, but they didn't take it. They had learned to be helpless. Turns out that rats and humans do the same.

Aaron Beck built on Seligman's learned helplessness theory but gave it a twist. He said depressed people have negative thoughts about themselves, the world, and the future.

- Self: low self-esteem comes from a belief that you are inadequate and of little value.

- World: seeing yourself as unable to experience pleasure.
- Future: believing things will not improve.

Adherents of this "cognitive model" say your worldview is colored by your thoughts. You know the score. Thoughts are deemed to influence symptoms of depression as well as your actions and attitudes. Negative thinking creates low moods.

There's much more about Freud's psychodynamic model in IDEA 39, *Get off the couch*. IDEA 27, *It's the thought that counts*, and IDEA 49, *Shades of gray*, will give you more about cognitive approaches.

Try another idea...

SOCIAL MODEL

Social scientists have developed the so-called social model: Depression is believed to be triggered by things going on in your life that may appear to be unconnected. Subscribers of the social model argue people may become and remain depressed due to societal influences. Your social class, job, and role in society can all be triggers. Sociologist George Brown and psychiatrist Tirril Harris identified several vulnerability factors for women that increased the likelihood of depression, namely no employment outside the home, the lack of a confiding relationship, having several young children at home, and losing her mother at an early age.

PSYCHODYNAMIC MODEL

Sigmund Freud introduced the world to his psychodynamic model: Your subconscious mind and early childhood experiences are responsible for present patterns of feelings and behavior. He suggested susceptibility to depression comes from early experiences of real or imagined loss. This approach is like foie gras: people either love it or hate it.

"Your theory is crazy, but it's not crazy enough to be true."
NIELS BOHR

Defining idea...

How did
it go?

Q **I've been told by various people that genetic predisposition, my acrimonious divorce, and chemical imbalances have caused my depression. These different approaches seem a bit disparate. How can they all be right?**

A *Try thinking of them as different perspectives on depression, with none telling the whole story. The root cause of depression is usually a combination of vulnerability, triggering, and maintaining factors.*

Q **My doctor's approach is very biological, with different drugs all the time. I'm out of work and on my own and am sure that this contributes to my moods. Can you suggest someone who'll work using the social model?**

A *Ask to see an occupational therapist. Their focus on employment and recreational activities may be closer to what you're looking for.*

Q **I asked my therapist what model she was using and she said she was an eclectic practitioner. What does this mean?**

A *Some of us don't feel an allegiance to one or other school of thought. We pick and mix from different models to treat specific problems. Most of us have strong influences though and your therapist might be prepared to talk about these to help you understand where she's coming from.*

26

The best-laid plans

We all dream. But when you're depressed, dreams seem to stay out of reach. Find out how expecting the best will bring out your best.

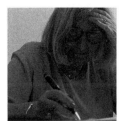

Planning for the good life could make this year the year when all your dreams come true.

If you expect the worst, you'll act in ways that ensure it comes true. Not convinced? Take Charlotte. She was fed up with being single, but didn't believe she'd ever meet anyone. She didn't bother with the way she looked and barely contributed to conversations, as she thought she'd bore people. One year she resolved to meet a partner. She had a makeover, started going out, and made a massive effort to be more chatty and sociable. John thinks he'll never get a job. Half the time he plans on sending off application forms, but doesn't get around to it before the closing date. When he does fill them in, he does it halfheartedly and the few times he's been interviewed he's underperformed.

People who plan get to anticipate and decide what they want and get from life, rather than just reacting to events and playing catch-up. Ready to try it? Great. Fast-forward twelve months and imagine how you'd like your life to be. Not how you think things might turn out, but how you'd like your life. Ask yourself what you

Here's an idea for you... **Start a motivational notebook or binder of ideas that support your goal. If you're trying to lose weight, you might start a collection of low-fat recipes. Paste in pictures of people you admire, or friends and relatives who support you. Next time you read an inspiring article, quote, or poem, stick it in. Once a month, review your monthly goals. Reading through your notebook will spur you on to success.**

want. Maybe you want to get back to work, or to get ahead in your career. Perhaps you want to be a better parent or return to college. Many people plan to make more time for themselves.

Once you know what you want to achieve, you're ready to set targets for the year ahead. These three tips will help you set effective goals:

1. Phrase each goal in a positive, upbeat way. To eat three healthy, balanced meals a day is better than "to stop stuffing my fat face with more junk."

2. Be specific. When you set your goal, some self-imposed deadlines give you something tangible to work toward.

3. Stick it to the wall. Or on the fridge, in fact anywhere you'll see and be reminded of it. Writing goals down makes them more powerful and it's more likely that you'll achieve them.

Once you've made a list of goals, choose the three most important ones. If you're struggling, think about which areas of your life, such as family, friends, job, riches, education, and spirituality, are most important to you. Have another look at these three, making sure

If you're struggling to fit everything into your busy schedule, then IDEA 7, *The time of your life*, shows you how to get back hours every week.

Try another idea...

that they'll bring about the life you imagined in the exercise above. They'll help you take small steps toward realizing your dreams. Their unique combo of short-term motivation and long-term vision helps you concentrate on what really matters and can stop you from getting distracted. Your self-confidence, which has probably taken a bashing recently, will be boosted as you start to achieve your goals and feel more in control of your destiny.

Next, set twelve smaller monthly goals that'll help you reach your yearly goal. For example, if your yearly goal is to move to a bigger apartment, your first monthly goal might be meeting with your accountant to find out how much you can afford. Your second monthly goal could be putting your current home on the market, followed by, in the third month, signing up with six real estate agents. Weekly and daily to-do lists help you break your monthly goal into manageable stages.

"Always shoot for the moon. Even if you miss you'll land among the stars."
LES BROWN, singer

Defining idea...

How did
it go?

Q **I used to be a long-distance runner, but after the kids were born I got very depressed and started comfort eating. I'm out of shape and overweight. Last year I promised myself I'd get fit and be able to do the New York marathon. Three months in, it seemed hopelessly unrealistic and I gave up the gym and put the weight I'd lost back on. I'm determined to try again. How can I avoid failure this time?**

A *It doesn't sound as if you've failed. You were able to lose weight and get fitter and it sounds as if you're more determined than ever. You may not have achieved your goal, but there is a lot you can learn from it. The first lesson is to be a little more realistic this time around. It may be better taking a longer-term view and going for the full marathon in, say, three years' time, working toward a half-marathon eighteen or twenty months from now. On a Post-it note, write down how you'll feel when you run the marathon and stick this to the treadmill when you train. If you imagine every step you take bringing you one step closer to that feeling, you'll be less likely to give up after a bad day or two.*

Q **I did a year planner but only achieved two of my goals. Where did I go wrong?**

A *I don't think you did. When you're depressed, it's easy to give yourself a hard time and ignore what's gone well. Go out and celebrate your achievements. It sounds as if you're well on the way to even better things.*

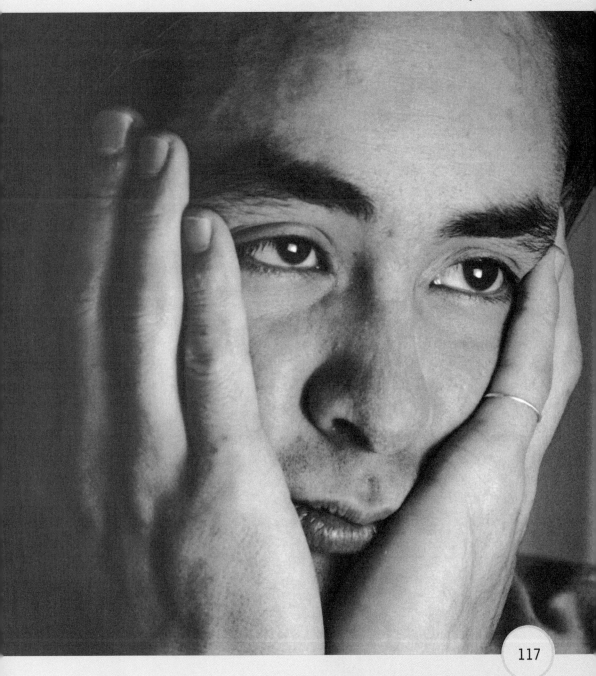

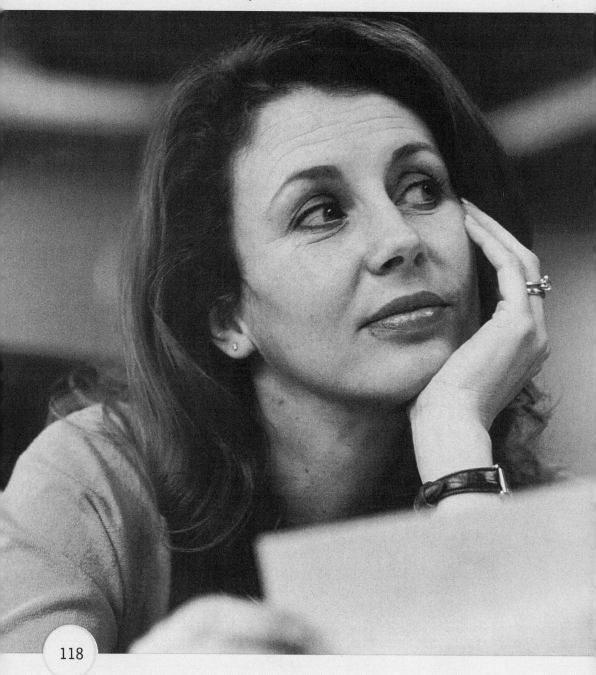

27

It's the thought that counts

Do you tend to jump to the wrong conclusions? Stress not, we've all done it. But learning to avoid it could be key to your recovery.

Replacing incorrect assumptions with reality testing can quash depression. It's easier than you think.

LOOK BEFORE YOU LEAP (TO THE WRONG CONCLUSION)

Our thoughts and feelings are interconnected. I was reminded of this the other day when I was walking by a river. Suddenly, a man pushed me off the path. I was frightened, thinking I was about to be mugged. Within a second, I realized he'd pushed me out of the way of a racing rollerblader, out of control and unable to stop. My feelings turned to gratitude when I realized I'd been spared a collision. When I thought of his push as a rescue attempt, not a threat, my feelings changed. But what's this got to do with defeating depression?

Everyone jumps to conclusions sometimes, but in depression our conclusions are often inflexible, self-blaming, and just totally off-track. Perhaps the woman you like on the bus won't look you in the eye so it proves you're doomed to propping up the singles bar forever. Or maybe your boss pointed out a small mistake and now you think she wants to fire you because you're useless. Because you feel bad about

Here's an idea for you...

Dedicate a day to practice different ways of seeing things. Whenever something happens, catch yourself from jumping to conclusions by asking yourself if there are any other ways of seeing it.

yourself, these guesses might seem believable, but they're wrong. More likely the woman on the bus is shy, or your boss thinks your work is great apart from one teensy error. When you react rather than think things through, miserable feelings frequently follow. You're more likely to miss out on life's good side, leading to more dollops of depression.

JILTED JULIE

It's scary when you see how quickly one bad thought leads to another. Julie was waiting for her husband, Neil, to pick her up from the airport after a long weekend with friends. Everyone else's partner was there, many with big bunches of flowers, but Neil didn't show. Instead of being annoyed, Julie felt terribly dejected, unloved, and unlovable. Here's how her thoughts escalated in just a few seconds:

> Neil hasn't come to get me.
> This is because he has forgotten.
> He is probably watching football on TV.
> If Neil really loved me, he'd be here.
> All my friends have been picked up, which proves they are better than me.
> Neil doesn't care about me. He cares more about football.
> Neil obviously hasn't missed me or he'd be here.
> I'll never have a happy relationship like all my friends have.
> Nobody loves me.
> I'll always be lonely.
> What's the point?

Whoa. See how thoughts can spiral out of control? Maybe Julie's right and Neil is at home with his feet up, but are there any other explanations?

> Neil's stuck in traffic.
> He's in a car crash.
> He forgot.
> He mixed the dates up.

Why go it alone? Noticing and challenging wrong conclusions needn't be a solitary activity. Check out IDEA 45, *I'll be there for you*, to find out how friends can support you.

Try another idea...

When we're depressed, we need to ditch rapidly drawn conclusions and opt instead for a reality check. So, if the washing machine floods your kitchen, you might think "The whole house is in chaos." But the reality check would be something like this: "I've got a lovely home. The kitchen's flooded, but it's only water and nothing's been damaged. I can call someone to repair the machine and it will be fixed. Of course I'm going to feel frustrated but there's no need for me to blow it out of proportion."

"Men are not defined by things but by the view they take of them."
EPICTERUS

Defining idea...

Next time you jump to a conclusion, ask yourself these four questions:

1. How would this seem to me if I wasn't depressed?
2. How would other people see this situation?
3. What alternative explanations are there?
4. Does my conclusion fit the facts?

"There is neither good nor ill, but thinking makes it so."
WILLIAM SHAKESPEARE, *Hamlet*

Defining idea...

Finally, ask yourself if other people agree with it. If you've got it wrong, it's time to change your conclusion. Which is what Julie did when it turned out Neil was at the airport, just at the wrong terminal.

How did it go?

Q **This reality testing sounds too simple. I just can't see it working for me. Any ideas to change my mind?**

A *Sounds like a wrong conclusion to me. Instead, try a reality check by asking yourself, "What have I got to lose?"*

Q **I've tried reality testing and it works, but only up to a point. Whenever I have a bad day, I end up feeling that all this thought challenging is just another fad and doomed to failure. Can you help?**

A *It's tough trying this stuff out. Getting the hang of thinking differently when you're depressed is really difficult. When you recover from depression, it doesn't happen overnight. Instead, most people find they start having good days and gradually these outnumber bad days. Next time you have a bad day, could you try seeing your setback as a chance to practice reacting to unhelpful thoughts? I found doing this encourages more helpful thinking.*

Q **I was brought up to believe that you should always listen to your gut reaction, and now you're saying those thoughts could be wrong. How can I know what to think?**

A *Everyone makes snap judgments and they are often right. Trouble is, when you're depressed your first thoughts about a situation are likely to be rigid and self-blaming, and these are often wrong and make you even more miserable. I'm not suggesting you ignore all your gut reactions, just do a little reality testing and see if they measure up.*

28

Let them all talk

If you're looking for a potent talking treatment, working it out with fellow sufferers could be the answer.

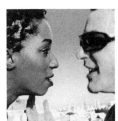

You know how peer pressure persuades kids to do things their mothers never dreamed possible? Group therapy can do the same for people with depression.

CONFESSIONS OF A GROUP GROUPIE

Group therapy is amazingly powerful. This might sound like the spiel of a pushy door-to-door saleswoman, but it's changed my life completely. How? Groups work because you're helped by people who know how you feel. The sense of isolation that brands depression doesn't stand a chance when facing a dozen others who've been through something similar or worse. These people aren't stuffed full of book knowledge; they've been there. And if you have to pay for therapy, group therapy is generally cheaper than individual sessions.

Here's an idea for you... **Check out some virtual group therapy. Online communities can offer similar benefits, are there when you need them, and save you bus fare.**

WHO'S TALKING NOW?

In group therapy, encouragement, advice, and constructive criticism are proffered by other people with depression as well as by therapists. Self-help groups are different from therapy groups since they're run by and for people with depression. Both types of groups can stop you from feeling isolated, as you'll see your circumstances, thoughts, and feelings aren't unique. Either way, you'll be able to share painful experiences, strong feelings, coping skills, and know-how, as well as seek out and give advice.

Free from professional constraints, fellow patients are often brutally honest. Comments like "You couldn't even kill yourself properly," may be hard to hear, but they drag you out of a self-pitying rut, forcing you to confront ambivalent feelings about living and dying.

REACH OUT

Listening to others' experiences often puts our problems into perspective. Helping people can be hugely rewarding, while hearing alternative suggestions enables you to see the world through other people's eyes.

WHAT'S GOING ON?

Understanding a bit about group dynamics helps you make sense of difficult meetings. It's said that groups go through these four stages:

Forming: In newly formed groups, people are generally on their best behavior; members get to know each other and build up trust.

Storming: Once the niceties are out of the way, things often heat up. Participants usually start to feel pissed off with each other and you might find yourselves competing to speak and be heard. Arguments abound and lots of people are tempted to sulk off. But it isn't all bad, as you'll learn to stomach confrontation and acquire invaluable arbitration skills.

Norming: Roles and relationships get established. You'll feel a strong sense of "being in the same boat" and a culture will emerge. You can tell this has happened when the same person is always five minutes late, or a certain someone always has to have the last word.

Performing: Down to business. Groups in this stage work together to make decisions, problem-solve, and support one another.

Try another idea...

Sometimes group therapy touches on topics you'd rather figure out one-on-one. You might need to invest in some individual attention. IDEA 3, *Docs, shrinks, and quacks*, points you in the right direction and saves you from charlatans.

Defining idea...

"My routines come out of total unhappiness. My audiences are my group therapy."
JOAN RIVERS

GATHER A GANG

No local group? Perhaps you could start your own using these five steps:

1. Plan, plan, plan
Decide who your group is for and what you hope to achieve. Where will you meet? How often? How will you let people know about the group? What ground rules are important? Will you provide refreshments? Who's going to foot the bills?

2. Don't go it alone
It's impossible to overstate the importance of finding some like-minded souls to set up a new group with you. Sharing roles and responsibilities is fundamental.

3. Look and learn
It's often worth paying a one-off visit to a similar group. Speaking to the organizers and picking their brains can save you a lot of time and trouble.

4. Call the doctor
Even if you don't want professionals present, it's worth getting them on your side. They're often willing to advertise groups in their waiting rooms or to give presentations to your members.

5. Look after number one
At the risk of sounding patronizing, consider your health. Are you well enough to take this on? Could starting a group make you worse?

Q **I'd like to join a group, but I don't know where to start looking. Where can I find out more?**

A *Your doctor should be able to tell you about therapy groups in your neighborhood. Libraries and national depression organizations will have lists and contact details of local self-help groups.*

Q **How long does group therapy take?**

A *This varies. Many groups are time-limited, typically running between twelve and twenty weeks, but others may be more open-ended, with different people starting and moving on over the years.*

Q **The thought of baring my soul to hordes of strangers fills me with horror. Any way around this?**

A *Joining a group can be intimidating, but remember, everyone else was new once and will make you welcome. You'll need to be a bit brave but it's worth it. It's unlikely you'll face dozens of people, as groups generally have between six and ten members, plus a therapist or two. Nobody will make you stand up and talk about stuff you'd rather keep to yourself.*

How did it go?

127

Q   **I think group therapy would be a good way to meet a guy who really understands what I've been through. My friend says relationships are banned in therapy groups. Is she right?**

A   *It depends on the group. Some are strict and don't allow any contact between meetings, others encourage you to make friends. Having a relationship with another group member can be a bad idea because you run the risk of either upsetting people with your loved-up smugness or airing all your dirty laundry if things go badly. People do meet in therapy, but planning to use a group as a sort of dating agency sounds like a recipe for disaster.*

29
Just say no

Are you a people pleaser? Can't say no, so you overcommit yourself? It's time to learn the art of polite refusal and show depression the door.

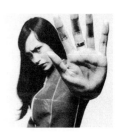

Fed up with being taken for granted? It's hard to say no when you feel pitiful or worthless. Maybe you feel that you have no control over what happens. The snag is, helplessness feeds depression.

If you're a people pleaser, you'll know that if you always say yes to others, you're soon taken for granted. Learning to say no puts you back in control and stops feelings of powerlessness. When I was newly qualified, I got piqued when colleagues assumed I'd do other doctors' jobs as well as my own. It took me a while to figure out that I'd set this up by beaming and obliging every time I was asked, "While you're here, could you just…?" Saying yes seemed like a good idea, but by being eager to make a good impression, I turned myself into a doormat. I've since learned that saying no doesn't mean I'm snubbing people, just that I'm declining demands.

Here's an idea for you...

Next time someone makes a request that you're not sure about, ask for time to think about it. When the pressure's off, it'll be easier to call or write to explain you'd like to, but just can't fit it in right now.

...and another idea

If you've been talked out of previous refusals, try starting sentences with the word "No." It's harder to backtrack if it's the first word you say.

Defining idea...

"The art of leadership is saying no, not saying yes. It is very easy to say yes."
TONY BLAIR

POLITE REFUSALS

When you say no, keep it short and stick to your point. Here are some nice ways of saying no:

- *Let's go for a swim.*
  Sorry, I really don't enjoy swimming.

- *Why don't you copy my essay?*
  That's really sweet of you, but I want to do my own work.

- *Want to come back for coffee?*
  No, I can't stay out late, I've got an early start tomorrow.

- *Let's meet at the gym after work.*
  I'd really rather not go to the gym today.

- *Why don't you come to the sales with me?*
  Maybe you'd better ask someone else; shopping isn't my idea of fun.

Try using body language to back up what you say. Shaking your head while saying no is a good start. And avoid changing your mind, however much demanding, imploring, or flattery you face. In time you'll become skilled at not only saying no, but saying no without feeling guilty. I figure it took me about a year.

BEING NEIGHBORLY

My neighbor Tom was afraid of saying no to his older brother and roommate Max. Tom ended up doing lots of things for Max, like picking up his dry cleaning, and was annoyed at being treated like an errand boy. Max took Tom for granted, while Tom believed if he ever said no, he'd lose his brother's friendship. I persuaded Tom to do an experiment. Next time Max sent Tom to collect his dry cleaning, Tom politely said no, explaining he had better things to do on his lunch hour. Max was annoyed, but Tom realized it didn't do either of them any harm. Their relationship survived and Tom no longer feels spineless.

People often say yes because they want to be liked. IDEA 17, *On top of the world*, gives you better ways of boosting your self-esteem.

Try another idea...

I'D LOVE TO BUT . . .

Still squirming at the thought of saying no? Take a leaf out of Jessie's book. Jessie's a champion cake baker. She's also a teacher and single mom of three. Lots of people ask Jessie if she'll bake a cake for charity cake sales, birthdays, and weddings. In the past, she always said yes, often staying up late and getting up ridiculously early to get the baking or decorating finished. A hobby that had been the source of so much pleasure started to stress her out. Now when she's asked to bake, she sighs and says, "You know, I'd really love to, but, I've just got too much to do. Maybe next time." If you're uneasy about an outright no, how about presenting a trade-off like, "I might just be able to do that, if you babysat for me/cleaned my car/did my shopping."

"You'd worry less about what others thought of you if you knew how seldom they do it."
OLIN MILLER, writer

Defining idea...

How did it go?

Q **I'm uncomfortable with saying no because it sounds so aggressive. How can I get around this problem?**

A *It can, but it depends how you say it. I agree that saying something like, "No way. I'd never get involved with anything like that," is aggressive, but you could make a more assertive comment like, "Sorry I can't help you out with that. I've already got plans for Saturday."*

Q **A lot of the time I say yes and only realize afterward that I should have said no. I take on too much and then feel stressed and overwhelmed. What can I do?**

A *Don't lose heart. You're halfway there by realizing when it would be better to say no. Really saying no is difficult. Next time this happens, why not go back and say you've changed your mind. You'll probably feel mortified the first time you do it, and your friends may be shocked that you've let them down or gone back on your word. But you'll also feel relieved and more confident. Once these feelings outweigh your horror of saying no, it'll become second nature.*

30

Reboot the hard drive

Many people with depression misconstrue events or circumstances. Swapping negative spin for more levelheaded thinking changes your mood.

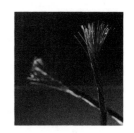

What you think about what's happening affects the way you feel.

"I'm a terrible artist," says Funmi. "People just buy my work because they feel sorry for me. None of my pictures ever turn out right."

"My husband's heart attack is my fault," says Hamida. "I stress him out and now I won't be able to cope on my own while he's in the hospital."

"I've got to wear glasses," says Kieron. "I look so geeky, no one will ever like me again."

Ever have thoughts like these? If so, it's time to reboot your hard drive. When you're depressed, you're more inclined to see the worst in yourself, the world, and your future. This negative spin takes several guises:

- *Assuming the worst*
  My wife hasn't called. She must have been killed in a car crash on the way home from work.

Here's an idea for you... **Grab a pen and paper and jot down the last thing that left you feeling miserable. Now draw a line down the page, and on the left-hand side scribble a list of any negative spin you might have put on it. On the right, see if you can come up with a levelheaded thought to replace it. Finally, look at each item on both lists. How does each one make you feel? It takes a while to get the hang of this, but once you've had a few tries, you'll be a champion levelheader.**

■ *Assuming everything is going badly when only one thing has gone badly*
I failed that exam so there's no point in going to school tomorrow. I'll be unemployed forever.

■ *Focusing on the bad stuff, while ignoring the good stuff*
That novel I had published is bound to be remaindered because there's a typo on page fifteen.

■ *Putting a negative slant on everything positive*
My boss only gave me a good appraisal because he feels sorry for me.

IS YOUR GLASS HALF FULL?

Defining idea... **"If you never change your mind, why have one?"**
EDWARD DE BONO

Two friends, Melanie and Jill, had wildly different thoughts, leading to opposite reactions to the same situation. One Saturday, Elaine and Melanie went to a singles party. Elaine met a guy and was asked on a date. Melanie didn't. Melanie thought: *Elaine is prettier than me. I'll never get asked out. Nobody understands me. I am worthless.* She became depressed, which lasted for two weeks.

The following Saturday, Elaine and Jill went to a singles party. Elaine met another guy and was asked on a date. Jill didn't. Jill thought: *Elaine's been here before, she knows how to get a date. It'll be my turn next time. I didn't see anyone I liked anyway. I had fun dancing, even though I didn't meet anybody.* She was mildly disappointed, but got over it by Sunday afternoon.

If your thinking is closer to Melanie's than Jill's, learning to replace your negative spin with more realistic explanations is guaranteed to lift your mood.

SPIN DOCTORING

Swapping negative spin for more balanced thinking takes some practice. Ask yourself if you could be spinning in the way you are thinking. The trick is to balance every negative notion with a more levelheaded one.

Jumping to the wrong conclusions? Stress not, we've all done it. Learn how to avoid it in IDEA 27, *It's the thought that counts.*

Try another idea...

"This is my depressed stance. When you're depressed, it makes a lot of difference how you stand. The worst thing you can do is straighten up and hold your head high because then you'll start to feel better. If you're going to get any joy out of being depressed, you've got to stand like this."
CHARLIE BROWN

Defining idea...

135

Here's how Melanie attempted this exercise:

Melanie's thoughts on Saturday night	How she could have seen it
It's just as well I didn't get asked out. I would have blown it anyway.	It's not true that it would all go wrong. I won't know until I try.
I'm a loser.	I'm not a loser. I've got a good job, two lovely kids, four close friends, and a nice home.
I should stop going to these singles parties. I'm just wasting my time.	If I stop going out, I'm unlikely to meet anyone.
I'll never meet anyone.	I won't if I give up.
I'll be on my own forever.	I don't have to be alone. I can choose to keep meeting people until I find Mr. Right.

I'm sure you've heard the notion of a cup being half full or half empty as two different perspectives of the same thing. If you can try to rephrase thoughts to make them seem more optimistic, you'll make major inroads on your depression.

Q **It's fairly easy to make a list of my negative spin, but I find it difficult to come up with alternatives. How can I generate more?**

How did it go?

A *This can be a difficult exercise and it's great that you've started. Have you thought about sharing your list with a good friend or relation? Asking someone who isn't depressed, "What do you think?" can be a good way of breaking out of a well-established spin.*

Q **I hate those people who put on a false air of optimism. It never seems to ring true. Isn't it better to be true to myself, even if it means staying miserable?**

A *As the old adage goes, laugh and the world laughs with you, cry and you cry alone. Clearly it's important to be true to yourself, but by giving in to negative spin, you're doing yourself a massive disservice, as there's a real chance you'll exacerbate your depression.*

Q **How can I be sure that my alternatives are really more levelheaded and not just more negative spin?**

A *It can be hard to tell the difference at first, especially if you've been stuck in a depressed mind-set for a long time. Try checking your new ways of seeing things with a friend, relative, or therapist or asking them how they would see things. Nobody else around? A quick and easy way to tell is to ask yourself how it makes you feel. If it doesn't make you feel any better, chances are it's more spin.*

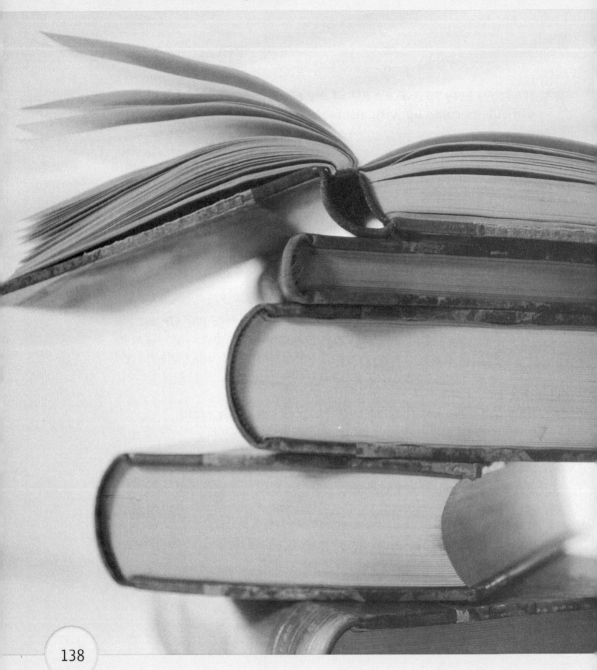

31

A novel idea

Lost the plot? Instead of ruminating about how miserable you feel, get reading. Find out about four books that can help you toward that elusive happy ending.

Ever wished you could just get away from it all? Pick up a book and you can. Good books introduce you to new countries, time zones, and mind-sets.

Stuck in a rut? Books offer new ideas and possibilities. Reading can also help you lose yourself for a few hours. Escaping into well-written prose is often comforting and relaxing.

AS OTHERS SEE US

Reading, it goes without saying, predates cinema and television, let alone other forms of mass communication. Bookworms would claim reading has virtues superior to other forms of entertainment. How many books can you think of that were better than the film or TV series? The people and locations you conjure up in your imagination from an author's abstract ink markings are generally better than even the best director. Books, whether a nineteenth-century classic or a contemporary thriller, are so plentiful that in ten lives you could only skim the surface of what's out there.

Here's an idea for you... **Start a book club or reading group—you'll be able to get rid of isolation, depression, and share ideas in one hit. Everyone reads the same book and meets monthly to discuss it. All you need is about six or seven other people with depression and some questions as conversation starters to get going. Advertise at your local library, community mental health clinic, general practitioner, or bookstores. Selecting a regular night makes it easier for people to stick to it and plan around other commitments.**

I could rave about Dickens' *A Tale of Two Cities*, *Pride and Prejudice* by the divine Jane Austen, or the work of modern greats like John Updike, but I won't. For the purpose of this idea I've restricted my recommendations to four books that tackle the thorny subject of mental illness. Without giving away any of the plots, all these texts are aspirational and ultimately uplifting. They offer succour and hope to even the most jaded and despairing reader.

Prozac Nation: Young and Depressed in America—A Memoir, by Elizabeth Wurtzel

In her psychologically powerful self-portrait, Elizabeth Wurtzel rips to shreds well-meaning but exhausted friends, toxic parents, and ineffectual therapists hiding behind professional personas. "What on earth makes a woman in her mid-twenties, thus far of no particular outstanding accomplishment, have the audacity to write a three-hundred page volume about her own life and nothing more, as if anyone else would actually give a shit?" she asks in her afterword. Some say she's a spoiled, self-indulgent whiner; others identify with her and hang on to every word. For my money, this is a fantastic account of what it's really like to be in and out of the pit of despair for a decade and come out alive. Aching, heartrending, but she gets there in the end.

Asylum, by Patrick McGrath

This story, set in a secure hospital in the 1950s, is a gripping account of love, obsession, institutions, and mental illness. Stella, a psychiatrist's wife, feels uncared for and her ambition is thwarted. She falls madly in love with one of her husband's inpatients. *Asylum*, though a dark and disturbing read, instills hope and is a good antidote to pessimism. If nothing else, the haunting beauty of his prose will distract you from your distress. It will probably do much more than that.

If all that reading has got your creative juices flowing, then doing some writing of your own can be therapeutic. Find out how in IDEA 4, *Dear diary*.

Try another idea...

The Bell Jar, by Sylvia Plath

This harrowing and insightful diary of depression is definitely worth a look. Talented Esther Greenwood, heroine of Sylvia Plath's autobiographical novel, becomes profoundly depressed while working as an intern on a fashion magazine. She attempts suicide, is admitted to a psychiatric hospital and following treatment she feels the "bell jar" of depression lifting. As the books ends, Esther is getting ready to leave the hospital and considers herself changed for the better.

An Unquiet Mind, by Kay Redfield Jamison

Professor Kay Redfield Jamieson is one of my heroes. She's an international authority on manic depression, a condition she also suffers from. *An Unquiet Mind* is an intelligent, articulate account of her destructive low moods, catastrophic spending sprees, relationship breakdowns, and suicide attempt. She tries to resolve heartrending but important questions like: "Which of my feelings are real?" and "Which of the me's is me?" This is a book to be inspired and encouraged by.

"To read a writer is for me not merely to get an idea of what he says, but to go off with him and travel in his company."
ANDRÉ GIDE

Defining idea...

How did it go?

Q **It's hard to find time to read. I'm also a very slow reader. How can I fit it in?**

A *Have you considered reading on the move? Try carrying a book around with you and dipping into it every time you're waiting, say, at the bus stop, in the supermarket, or on the train. You could also try reading instead of watching TV. I like reading before going to sleep at night. My husband, a literary critic, often reads during the night if he can't sleep or first thing when he wakes up.*

Q **I find it really difficult to concentrate. Any suggestions?**

A *Try something light. The Sunday papers are a better starting point than the collected works of Shakespeare. Compilations of short stories or poems are good places to develop your concentration before moving on to novels or biographies with short chapters.*

Q **I've always been a bookworm and used to enthuse about what I'm reading. But since I got depressed, other people's sneering makes me feel worse. They seem to think I'm trying to be more educated and brainier than I am, but I just love books and reading. Can you help?**

A *Why not join a reading circle or book club where everyone reads the same book and talks about it? It will also put you in touch with other bookworms who won't make you feel like a fish out of water. If there isn't one nearby you could try one online.*

32

Rant and rave

Anger management might sound like soft-core therapy for thugs, but its effects can be dramatic. It isn't getting angry that's the problem, it's how you express it.

Anger's a potentially useful emotion, but how to deal with it? Learning how to transform rage into passion helps you gain advantage rather than lose it.

Depression stops you from doing things. It drains away motivation, drive, and energy. Anger, on the other hand, induces and even compels us to action. A former colleague saw her life's mission as making depressed people angry for this exact reason. Sigmund Freud went one further and thought depression is anger turned inward against yourself.

Do you worry about what would happen if you really lost it? Many people are scared that an angry outburst will ruin a relationship irretrievably. Acting in the heat of the moment means you are more likely to be impulsive or rash. Nobody wants to be a bully, so learning to calm down and channel your anger helps you use it in a positive way.

Here's an idea for you...

Over the next few weeks, each time you get angry spend some time afterward seeing if you can identify any common triggers. Discovering what or who presses your buttons means you can deal with anger in a more constructive, less destructive way.

BOILING OVER

Let's say you take a faulty teakettle back to the store. The store assistant is rude and refuses a refund. You ask for the manager. It's his day off. How do you respond? Maybe you feel angry, but lack the confidence to do anything about it. If you feel like this, chances are you'll go home without a replacement teakettle, feel bad and angry with yourself, and feel that life isn't fair. You might feel full of self-loathing for your inaction. Alternatively, you might get really angry. A furious and ugly shouting scene gets you evicted from the store, but probably won't get you a new kettle. But keeping your cool in the store, perhaps by counting to ten, and channeling your anger into a letter of complaint to the manager, will probably get you a new kettle.

If you're angry with the snotty kids who keep vandalizing the bus stop outside your house, getting angry can be helpful. Instead of charging out there and getting a criminal record for assaulting them, use your rage constructively. Get a neighborhood watch going. Organize a petition for CCTV at the bus stop. Get the local paper interested and campaign for an after-school club to keep bored kids off the streets.

Next time you feel your blood about to boil over, walk away and try these three techniques:

IDEA 29, *Just say no*, helps you come up with assertive rather than aggressive responses to people who rile you.

Try another idea...

1. Count to ten

I expect your dad taught you this one, but it's still got a lot going for it. Not only does it give you some essential cooling off time, it also distracts you temporarily, which can help give you a sense of perspective. It takes most people longer than thirty seconds to fully calm down though. Twenty minutes is a lot more like it, so be prepared to count to ten a few times or do something else for a while.

2. Pretend you're sitting opposite the person who's made your blood boil

Let rip and tell them what's on your mind. Now sit in their chair and imagine what your rant sounded like. Can you see it from their perspective? Instead of thinking, "Spencer's trying to piss me off," think "Spencer must be tired." If you can do this, you're more likely to respond in an assertive rather than aggressive way. What's the difference? Being assertive means standing up for yourself rather than attacking or hurting others. Rather than being loudmouthed or belligerent, reply in a firm but self-confident style.

3. Write a letter to the person you're angry with

Dump your inhibitions and say exactly how you feel. Be as abusive as you like. Then either burn or tear the letter up. Wait for a week and then write a more measured, conciliatory letter that you can mail.

"Heat not a furnace for your foe so hot that it do singe yourself."
WILLIAM SHAKESPEARE, *Henry VIII*

Defining idea...

Are you feeling calmer? Great. Now's the time to take action. Here's how:

1. Start sentences with an "I" statement

"I feel frustrated and let down because I was sold a faulty teakettle and wasn't given a refund" is better than "Your incompetent assistant was mean to me and refused to exchange your lousy kettle. You obviously lack judgment in your choice of staff, but I wouldn't have expected better from a cretin like you."

2. Describe things in a factual tone

In place of "Police waste so much time on stupid paperwork that I've had to take the law into my own hands," be specific: "I've written to Sergeant Plod to ask him to come see the damage done to the bus stop, but despite five phone calls I haven't received a response or an acknowledgement of my letter."

3. Say why you're angry

It might be obvious to you, but spelling it out means you're not dependent on other people's undeveloped mind-reading skills. "I feel angry because Sergeant Plod didn't come on Thursday as promised. Many residents were looking forward to hearing from him at the neighborhood watch meeting, which we have sadly had to postpone again."

Q   **All the anger-management techniques sound very good in theory, but when I get angry, I can't stop and think, so I end up losing it and not using any of them. Is there a way around this?**

How did it go?

A   *Don't lose heart. All new things can be difficult, but practicing helps. Why not try these techniques out when you're calm? For instance, could you role-play a potentially argumentative circumstance with a friend or partner?*

Q   **I try to avoid getting angry and walk away from conflict. Isn't it better to bottle things up a little rather than risk major confrontations?**

A   *'Fraid not. Unexpressed anger affects your thinking and behavior, and may worsen physical problems. Instead of seeing anger as something to escape from or suppress, try seeing your anger as a warning sign of a practical or emotional vulnerability that needs you to act.*

Q   **Sometimes I get so upset and angry I end up smashing things. Counting to ten at times like that just doesn't do it. It's about as effective as adding an ice cube to a vat of boiling water. What can I do to calm down?**

A   *I agree that counting to ten won't take all the heat out of a destructive fury. When you're this wound up, you need to get physical, but instead of slinging the Ming, walk, or better yet run, outside for twenty minutes. As well as using up some spare adrenaline, physically getting away from whatever's riled you helps.*

147

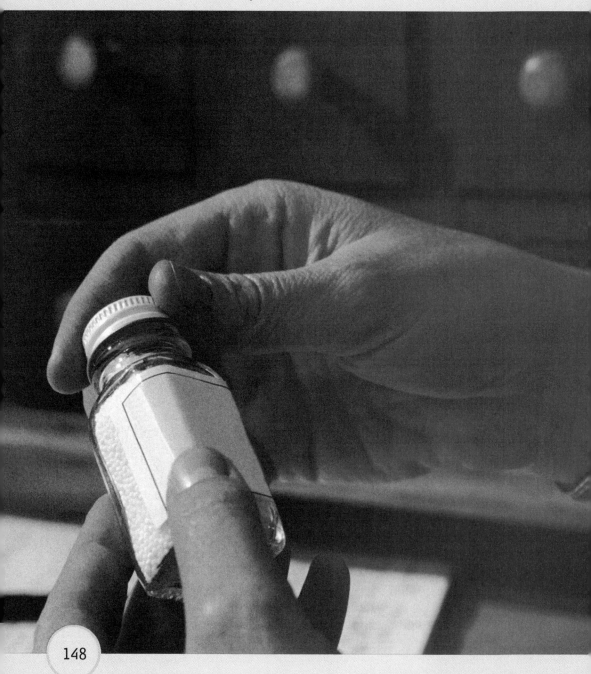

33

When the drugs don't work

About a third of people taking respectable doses of highly regarded antidepressants are still depressed one month later. What can you do if you're one of them?

Don't despair. You can still live (happily ever after) with treatment-resistant depression. Here's how.

No doubt you feel unhappy, tired, and don't enjoy the things you used to love doing, but there may be another explanation for your dejection. If you haven't found a way of dealing with depression, it may be time to revisit your original diagnosis.

HORMONES AND MOOD SWINGS

Miranda had been depressed for weeks and wasn't getting better. She felt slowed down, tired, her periods were irregular, she was constipated, and felt cold all the time. Miranda thought this was due to stress, but the real reason she wasn't getting better was because of a small gland at the front of her neck. We've all got one, it's called the thyroid gland, and its job is producing the hormones that regulate metabolism. Miranda had an underactive thyroid gland. Low thyroid hormone levels can cause awful depression that usually responds to thyroid hormone

Here's an idea for you... **If your treatment regime isn't working, make an appointment with your doctor and ask for a formal review of your diagnosis. This should include a physical examination and blood tests. Not happy? Why not seek out a second opinion or a specialist?**

replacement therapy. It's important to get thyroid hormone levels checked out so abnormalities are picked up and treated. Some people have low thyroid hormone levels but none of the bodily signs of thyroid disease. Vigorously correcting even borderline thyroid hormone levels has an immense effect on low mood.

VIRUS ALERT

Sienna's depression didn't get any better with treatment, either. She felt tearful and drained, but also had a sore throat she couldn't shake off. Her boyfriend noticed her eyes looked puffy, but they both thought it was because she had cried so much. Then her doctor did a blood test showing she had infectious mononucleosis, or glandular fever. This is a viral illness caused by the Epstein–Barr virus. As this got better, she stopped feeling so debilitated and dejected.

BIG D OR BIG C?

It was the first time Ernie had ever felt depressed. The pills and counseling didn't do much good. He lost his appetite and his clothes hung off him. After several weeks he turned yellow and his skin itched horribly. Ernie had pancreatic cancer. Pancreatic cancer doesn't cause any symptoms until it starts to spread. We think that people get depressed because the diseased pancreas causes chemical imbalances that lead to depression. I'm not trying to panic you. Most people with depression don't have cancer. Only around 10–20 percent of depression is set off by another illness, but it's important to rule out bodily causes for your low mood.

CLEAN BILL OF HEALTH

So you've been to the doctor and there's nothing else going on. Hand on heart time. Do you always take your medication? I know I often forgot. Are there things you could do to remind yourself, like crossing off a day on the calendar or putting a check in your schedule planner? Could you set up a daily reminder on your cell phone? Alternatively, you could invest in a compartmentalized pill container where you put in all the pills you have to take at particular times.

It's worth checking a couple of things out with your doctor:

- Am I on a high enough dose?
- Have I been on this dose for long enough to expect to notice an effect?

If it's a yes to both, it's probably time for a different drug. Antidepressants work in 70 percent of people. If you're one of the other 30 percent, you've got a 50/50 chance of busting your depression by changing antidepressants. I reckon it's worth a shot. If you're not yet having a regular talking treatment, there's never been a better time to get that going.

ESCALATE EFFECTS

If none of this helps, don't despair. The next step is trying something called augmentation. This means adding in another drug to make your antidepressant work better. There are a number of different drugs used for this, and they need to be properly tailored to your requirements by a professional.

Sounds wacky but a new magnetic treatment often works when other cures don't restore you to health. Check out IDEA 15, *Magnetic attraction*.

Try another idea...

"Reality is a crutch for people who can't cope with drugs."
LILY TOMLIN, actress

Defining idea...

151

CALL IN THE PRO'S PRO

If all else fails, ask for a referral to a specialist. Doctors and researchers spend their lives working out intricate treatment regimes. You could benefit from one of them and don't need to suffer in silence.

How did it go?

Q **I've heard about someone having brain surgery to cure depression. Does it work?**

A *You're referring to psychosurgery, a type of specialized brain surgery. It is used very rarely to treat depression that hasn't gotten better after numerous treatments have been tried for many months or years. It's a drastic step, doesn't work for everyone who has it, but can occasionally help when everything else has been exhausted.*

Q **I've been offered ECT because nothing else has worked for me. What do you think?**

A *Electroconvulsive therapy (ECT) is an incredibly effective treatment. It's probably the most powerful weapon in our depression-fighting armory. I've seen it be literally lifesaving, as it acts much more quickly than drugs. But, and it's a big but, many people who have had it say they have had lasting memory problems. Doctors have always been taught that patients might have a bit of forgetfulness around the time of ECT treatment, but I've heard too many contrary stories to believe this is the whole truth.*

34

Booze blues

You're stressed, miserable, and can't wait to curl up with a stiff drink. Here's how to avoid booze blues.

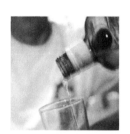

Everyone knows alcohol and misery can be a toxic combo. But should everyone with depression stay on the wagon?

You already know getting drunk makes you clumsy, slurs your speech, causes your stomach to cartwheel, makes you horny but unable to do much, and gives you monster hangovers. But, let's face it, drinking is also fun. It's how we relax, party, and escape life's problems. So it's understandable that you might have a drink to cheer yourself up, or to help you sleep.

Trouble is, alcohol messes with more than your mind. It scrambles brain chemistry, affecting circuits responsible for sadness, anxiety, poor sleep, and reduced appetite. So if you're a heavy drinker, drinking will make you depressed.

As well as making you miserable, alcohol makes you frustrated, irritable, angry, aggressive, paranoid, hopeless, and suicidal. It causes physical problems from hepatitis to stomach ulcers and impotence. And if that's not enough, it zaps your concentration, makes you forgetful, slows reaction times, jumbles thoughts, and causes permanent brain damage.

Here's an idea for you... **Try alternating soft and alcoholic drinks. This strategy may help you if you're finding it hard to stick to your limit.**

Too many benders can cause:

■ Permanent memory loss, a bit like Alzheimer's.
■ Psychosis: You'll start hearing voices.

■ Dependence: When you stop drinking, you get shaky, nervous, and seriously ill.
■ Suicidal feelings: Lots of people who want to kill themselves have alcohol problems. Most people who kill themselves have had a drink.

FEELING CAGEY?

At med school, we were taught to ask questions called CAGE—a contrived, but useful, acronym. Here's the score: Answer yes to more than two and you may be dependent.

C   Have you ever felt you should **cut** down your drinking?
A   Have people **annoyed** you by commenting on the amount you drink?
G   Have you ever felt **guilty** about your drinking?
E   Have you ever needed an **eye-opener** in the morning?

LAST ORDERS?

If you want to avoid all the toe-curling effects above, guys shouldn't drink more than fourteen drinks each week; women, seven drinks. To save you taking your home chemistry set out to dinner, use this handy list:

What's your tipple?	Serving
Glass of wine (out)	1
Glass of wine (home)	2
Glass of wine (home alone)	2½
Shot of spirits	1
Bottle of beer	1

Scared by this idea and pouring your third scotch? IDEA 35, *Doin' it differently*, will help you resist.

Try another idea...

You don't have to be a math whiz to see that if you're drinking every day, it doesn't take much to reach your limit.

DEAR DIARY...

It might make you cringe, but the only way you'll really know how much you drink is by keeping a diary. Rather than just writing down what you drink, use your diary to track other things affecting your drinking by answering: When? What? Where? Who was I with? Try to complete your diary while drinking; otherwise it'll be as useful as a shady government dossier. Dan's diary on the next page gives you the idea.

"I exercise strong self-control. I never drink anything stronger than gin before breakfast."
W. C. FIELDS

Defining idea...

155

Dan Dumbleweed's Drinking Diary

When	What	Where	Who
After work	2 beers	Fox and Hounds	With John and May
Before bed	3 big whiskeys	At home	Alone
Before work	Half bottle wine	Park bench	With local winos

At the end of each week, total up the drinks. Bar and restaurant measures tend to be pretty standard, but if you're like me, you'll be more generous when pouring yourself a drink at home, so play safe and assume your home drinks are worth double—unless you've been visiting an aunt who's stingy with her sherry.

CUTTING DOWN

Use your diary to identify potential trouble spots and come up with a game plan. I used to drink more out with work colleagues than non-work friends, so I cut down on after-work socializing. You could set yourself a limit, say, three alcoholic drinks. Continue with your diary and celebrate successes at the end of each week (not with a big bender). Don't be hard on yourself if you have a bad week. I'm not pretending I'm a Goody Two-shoes who orders a virgin version of Sex on the Beach every Saturday night. We all know we shouldn't drink too much, but, hey, occasional overindulgences happen to the best of us.

Try another idea... **Adrenaline and alcohol hit the same brain circuit. You'll be running from the bar and from depression after IDEA 40, *Pedal pushers*.**

Q **I've tried a drinking diary but it's not practical. I'd be laughed out of my local bar if I got my diary out, but when I try to write it down the morning after, I lose count. What can I do?**

How did it go?

A *Of course you want to keep your drinking diary to yourself. How about hiding it in your coat pocket and sneaking to the bathroom to update it at regular intervals? Only joking. You need a box of matches. There'll probably be some at the bar. Keep them in your pocket and every time you have a drink, break a match in half. The next day, you can count broken matches instead of relying on your memory. If you're not sober enough to break matches without your friends noticing, it's time to stop drinking.*

Q **A few days ago I gave up drinking but now I feel terrible. I'm edgy, can't sit still, and am scared, sweaty, and shaking. Why's this?**

A *Uh-oh. These sound like withdrawal symptoms. Because your body has gotten used to drinking, you need medical help to come off alcohol safely. Your doctor can give you medication like diazepam to stop these dreadful symptoms.*

Q **I drink heavily to blot out depression. I've tried to cut down but I'm not managing and am back up to about fifty drinks a week. Do you have anything for willpower?**

A *Setting goals is a bit of an art and several factors can mar your progress. The trick is to set a focused goal, like planning to cut down your drinking from fifty to forty-five drinks next week. Make it easier for yourself with an action plan. When are you drinking the most? Say it's on Saturday nights: Aim to cut that evening's drinking to twenty, tops, and try to have no more than three on other nights. With targets like this that are both reasonable and doable, it's a cinch.*

157

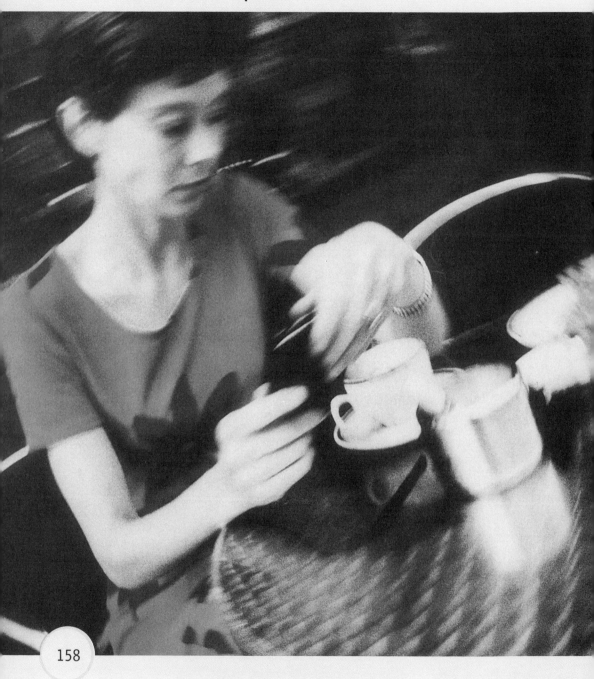

35

Doin' it differently

Scared of doing things differently? Here's your chance to experiment a little and turn self-fulfilling prophecies on their head.

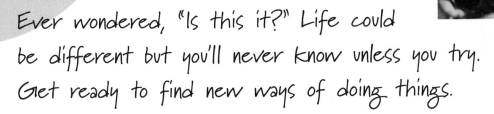

Ever wondered, "Is this it?" Life could be different but you'll never know unless you try. Get ready to find new ways of doing things.

Psychiatrists and other professionals use behavioral experiments to help patients find new ways of approaching old problems or attitudes. Pros use them to help people swap unhelpful ways of doing things for healthier actions. They're used to treat stress, panic, and depression. You become a sort of scientist, finding out what really happens if you do things differently.

Why the fuss? Once you've tried one you'll see they're a fast track to change. If you're looking for an idea that brings lasting changes, get your (lab) coat and see how Fareeda, Suzi, and Ned worked through this five-point plan:

1. What's your hunch? Use it to make a prediction.
2. Go over any supporting facts and see if you can find any evidence against it.
3. Devise an experiment to test your prediction.
4. What happens?
5. What does this mean?

Here's an idea for you...

Write down your experiments and their outcomes. This a great way to maximize what you learn and provides tons of inspiration for coping with hard times.

MEAL DEAL

Fareeda and Deepak are dentists. Their jobs are hectic and both work long hours, but Fareeda has a shorter journey home. She'd been cooking dinner every night for the two years they'd lived together and had started feeling tired and resentful. She tried the five-point plan.

Fareeda's forecast: "If I don't cook dinner tonight, Deepak will be angry when he gets in." What's her evidence? "I've cooked dinner every night and that's the way he likes it. I've managed to avoid making him angry so far; I'm scared to rock the boat." Could you design an experiment to test her forecast? Something like, "I won't cook tonight and will tell Deepak that I'm too tired."

Want to know what happened? Deepak didn't mind. He wasn't mad and took Fareeda out to dinner.

SUZI'S WRONG

Try another idea...

For added impact, IDEA 27, *It's the thought that counts*, helps you recognize and defy unhelpful thoughts feeding your depression.

Suzi believed if she refused a man sex on their first date, he'd get mad and wouldn't call her. She had a lot of one-night stands, but felt so used and dirty that she'd sneak out before the man woke up. The guy usually thought she didn't want to see him again, so didn't pursue things as a result. Suzi's relationships were doomed before they started. She decided to test her belief that men wouldn't call unless she had sex. Warren from Accounts asked Suzi for a drink after work. She accepted, had a fun evening, but got her own cab home. Did he call? You bet.

RETAIL THERAPY

When experiments don't go as planned, it's time to turn to IDEA 19, *I don't know what to do.* You'll find problem-solving strategies that will get you back on track.

...and another...

Ned's a serious shopaholic, a card-carrying member of Shopaholics Anonymous. He feels weak at the arrival of his monthly credit card bills and store card statements and dreads those visits from his loan shark. Ned's hunch? "If I don't buy things, I won't feel better." He thought about the evidence for this and said he got a real buzz out of buying stuff, but that this turned to guilt, worry, and dread when the bills started arriving. Ned came up with an experiment to test his hunch. He'd go to the stores, but leave his wallet at home. He thought window-shopping without buying would be disappointing, but it wasn't and he now enthuses about his guilt-free mood boost.

OVER TO YOU

Ready to give it a try? Great. Start by picking one of your hunches and plan an experiment to test alternatives. When you set up your experiment, ask yourself if it is practical and doable, so you avoid setting yourself up to fail. Make it as specific as you can, so you know exactly what you need to do. Next, try predicting the outcome. Pick a good time and do your experiment. What happens? How much does the outcome support your hunch?

"The person who says it cannot be done should not interrupt the person doing it."
CHINESE PROVERB

Defining idea...

161

How did
it go?

Q **I'm fed up with waiting on my boyfriend. The other night, I decided not to cook and he went ballistic. No candlelit dinner for me. What did I do wrong?**

A *Nothing. Experiments are about testing a theory and seeing what happens. While it is unpleasant to be with someone who "goes ballistic," there is always hope that the air could be cleared, resulting in your grievance having been heard and a chance you will no longer be taken for granted.*

Q **Everything always turns out badly for me, whatever I do. I'm sure I'm jinxed and can't see how these experiments could help. Can you convince me?**

A *When you're depressed, you tend to notice bad things or put a negative spin on stuff. Your gut feeling that there's no point trying this idea might be right, but say it isn't. Why settle for feeling ill-fated and miserable when there could be a way out? Why not give one of these experiments a try? Does it make a difference? You've got nothing to lose and my hunch is that feeling doomed and unhappy just won't cut it anymore. Only one way to find out.*

Q **I'm so depressed. I made a huge effort, got my hair cut, bought a new outfit, did my nails, the lot, and my partner didn't even notice. What should I do now?**

A *Find someone who appreciates you.*

36
Toil and trouble

Taking a sick day? Forget snuggling up for a dozen days in bed and discover the healing power of hard work.

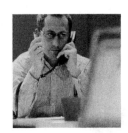

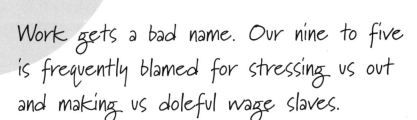

Work gets a bad name. Our nine to five is frequently blamed for stressing us out and making us doleful wage slaves.

Of course there's some truth in that, but we forget that nothing gives people a sense of nihilism faster than days doing nothing, staring into oblivion, hoping to become extinct. Here are ten reasons work works as a depression buster:

1. It raises self-esteem
2. It gives us a sense of purpose
3. Mastering a series of goals makes us feel good
4. We feel appreciated
5. It saves us from being social lepers and gives us an answer when people say, "And what do you do?"
6. It gives our days (and lives) structure
7. It's often a good place to make friends and hang out with them
8. It's a source of distraction from depressing thoughts
9. It's fun (sometimes)
10. It gives you choices

Here's an idea for you...

Grab a pen and paper and describe your dream job in as much detail as you can. Now imagine you're interviewing prospective candidates for your dream job. What are you looking for in the perfect candidate? Now imagine you're applying. Write or revamp your résumé. And try the interview questions. Would you give yourself the job? If not, what more do you need? What courses can you take? Who can help you?

MONEY TALKS

All right, I admit it, the money helps, too. Extra cash gives you control over your life and means you can make the sort of decisions you can't make on welfare—like "Barbados or St. Lucia?" When I was a medical student, I had a boyfriend who was unemployed. If you've been on welfare, you'll know all too well that without a paycheck, it's hard to plan ahead, you're dropped by society, and you're robbed of your identity.

WORK IT OUT

Now that you've decided to go, or go back, to work, there are things you can do once you're there that make it easier. Tell a trusted senior colleague you're feeling under par. They might be able to take some of the pressure off. When I was depressed, I found it hard to concentrate on written work, but could do mechanical things like making jewelery. If there are any physical jobs you could do instead of heavy-duty brain work, do it. Try to avoid hiding at your desk during lunch break. No matter if you like to chill out by the water cooler or cozy up with a cappuccino, chat to colleagues during breaks. Planning a weekly celebration for getting though another

Defining idea...

"It is impossible to enjoy idling thoroughly unless one has plenty of work to do."
JEROME K. JEROME

week will give you something to look forward to. Enjoy it, and your paycheck: You've earned both.

GETTING BACK TO WORK

What happens if you've been out of work for a long time and are anxious about getting back in the saddle? If you're employers are supportive, why not discuss a graded return with your boss? After being out sick for a long time, it makes sense for many people to go, say, three days per week initially, building up to full time over a couple of months. Many employers are happy to do this, as it retains employees rather than overburdening them and needing to pay out sick leave again. Alternatively, could you take on a little less responsibility for a couple of weeks until you get your confidence back? Either way, try returning on a Wednesday, as you won't have to face Monday morning pressures and you'll only have to work half a week before a weekend break.

Skip the over-boiled vegetables in the staff cafeteria and take a mood-boosting packed lunch to work. IDEA 21, *You are what you eat*, will whet your appetite.

Try another idea...

"Happiness does not come from doing easy work but from the afterglow of satisfaction that comes after the achievement of a difficult task that demanded our best."
THEODORE I. RUBIN, psychiatrist and author

Defining idea...

How did
it go?

Q **My wife's depressed and has a problem with work. She just can't stop. She's always at the office late, brings work home on weekends, and checks her email obsessively, even on vacation. That can't be good for her, can it?**

A *The phrase* work-life balance *comes to mind. Some people cope with depression by throwing themselves into their work, often destroying their health and families. See if you can encourage your wife to channel some of her time and effort into family activities.*

Q **I hate my job and feel like leaving. I'm tempted to resign, but I'm worried I won't get another job. I'm the main earner and we could lose our home if I'm unemployed. What would you do?**

A *Many people feel like walking out of jobs when they're depressed. I'm sure you have good reasons for hating work, but I'd strongly suggest you put off making major decisions like resigning until you're better. When you're depressed, you've probably got a lousy opinion of yourself, which means it's much harder to fill out applications and shine at interviews, preventing you from getting the sort of work you deserve. If you feel factors at work are making your depression worse, talking this through with occupational health therapists or your own doctor can be much more helpful than walking out.*

37

Cut it out

Cutting? Burning? Overdosing? If you're a self-harmer, here are some thoughts to help you through.

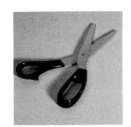

Some people hurt themselves to survive. Here's how to banish burns, limit damage, or quit cutting.

You might have heard some fancy names like deliberate self-harm, self-harm, self-mutilation, self-inflicted violence, self-cutting, parasuicide, and self-abuse. But I'm calling cutting, burning, taking overdoses, hitting yourself, banging your head against walls, and not letting wounds heal *hurting yourself*. Lots of people get these actions mixed up with suicide attempts, but the way I see it, hurting yourself is a way of coping with overpowering feelings that you can't express any other way.

If you hurt yourself, you don't need me saying it's a bad way of coping. You know this already, but sometimes things get out of control. Perhaps you've been blamed, uncared for, or badly treated by friends, family, or pros. For the record, if you hurt yourself, I don't think you're crazy, manipulative, or grotesque. I understand you don't choose to do it for attention and I know I've no right to insist you stop.

Here's an idea for you...

If you're not ready to stop cutting, then make it safer. When you're calm, decide how much hurt you'll allow yourself. You're aiming for the least amount of injury to take the edge off. Be specific. How many shallow cuts, superficial burns, whatever, will you make? Keep bandages nearby and learn to look after wounds. After you've cut, would it help to be with someone? If you choose to be alone, would it help to call someone?

CUTTING DOWN

Dr. Tracy Alderman, who knows lots about self-harm, suggests looking over these assertions if you're thinking about stopping. You don't need to be able to say yes to all, but the more yeses, the greater your chances of success:

- I have a solid emotional support system of friends, family, and/or professionals that I can use if I feel like hurting myself.
- There are at least two people in my life that I can call if I want to hurt myself.
- I feel at least somewhat comfortable talking about hurting myself with three different people.
- I have a list of at least ten things I can do instead of hurting myself.
- I have a place to go if I need to leave my house so as not to hurt myself.
- I feel confident that I could get rid of all the things that I might be likely to use to hurt myself.
- I have told at least two other people that I am going to stop hurting myself.
- I am willing to feel uncomfortable, scared, and frustrated.
- I feel confident that I can endure thinking about hurting myself without having to actually do so. I want to stop hurting myself.

If you want to stop, it helps to recognize and understand why you hurt yourself, so ask yourself: How do I feel before I hurt myself, and how do I feel afterward? Once you've understood why, give some of these alternatives a whirl.

I want to feel pain

Rub deep heat cream into your skin.

Squeeze ice cubes hard.

Instead of burning yourself, push an ice cube into your skin. It leaves a red mark and hurts but doesn't injure.

Wear an elastic band around your wrist and snap it.

Plunge your hands into a bag of frozen peas.

I hurt myself because I feel sad

It's time for some major pampering, so snuggle up with soothing music, a good book, and a warm drink. Fill your room with scented candles or go for an aromatherapy massage.

I hurt myself because I feel angry

Throw eggs or ice cubes against a garden wall.

Buy some cheap dishes in a secondhand shop and take out your rage with a hammer.

Slash, tear, or burn an old mail order catalog.

Smash up a coconut or pulp a melon.

I cut to see blood

If you feel like cutting your arms, draw around them and use a red pen to mark cuts you'd like to make. Or take this further: Strip, get in the shower, and scribble on yourself with red pen or lipstick. Dribble strawberry ice cream topping over places you'd like to cut. Dragging the nozzle over your arms almost mimics cutting.

Try another idea…

If you're addicted to cutting because of the buzz you get afterward, you'll find that exercise is a terrific way of getting a similar high. Check out IDEA 40, *Pedal pushers*.

Defining idea…

"When I was younger, I did self-mutilate. I'd be upset and it would calm me down…Sometimes the idea of self-destruction is very romantic. I got over that."
CHRISTINA RICCI, actress

169

How did it go?

Q **This probably sounds crazy, but I'm addicted to picking scabs. I cut myself every couple of weeks, but can't leave the scabs alone. There's something about sliding my finger under the crusts that has me hooked. Any tips?**

A *I don't think you're crazy. Go to your nearest Asian supermarket and buy henna. It comes in little tubes with a narrow nozzle. Instead of cutting, draw flowers, birds, or butterflies, using the nozzle as a pen. Leave it for twenty-four hours and over the next few days pick henna off like scabs. Your body art will fade over a couple of weeks.*

Q **Our daughter cuts her arms. We want to help but just don't understand why she does it. Can you explain it for us?**

A *When people hurt themselves, it's so frightening for parents, who often feel powerless and angry. The most important thing you can do is show your daughter you care. People hurt themselves for many reasons. Some say it's their way of dealing with overpowering feelings. Many people say they do it to feel alive and get rid of numbness. You can also help by suggesting she speak to a pro, as it's often a way of expressing feelings that are difficult to put into words.*

38

I did it my way

Fallen out with your doctor or therapist? Feeling ignored? These negotiation and conflict-resolution skills help you work with pros, even when you disagree.

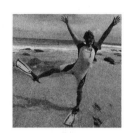

Regrettably, like all relationships, your dealings with helpers and healers can go hideously wrong.

I've been lucky enough to meet scores of professionals anyone would respect and admire. But I've also come across my share of boorish, emotionally gauche, and downright odd ones. And, I'm ashamed to say, there have been times I've fouled up, and I'm grateful to patients who took the trouble to set me straight.

TECHNICALLY SPEAKING

Experts Ellen Annandale of the UK's University of Warwick and Kate Hunt of the Medical Research Unit in Glasgow identified four types of disagreements between patients and health pros. Identify what's gone wrong and you're halfway to fixing it:

Disputes over the diagnosis: If you feel it's taken too long to get a depression diagnosis or you've been given a label you disagree with, try asking how they got to that conclusion. Ask yourself if there's any information that has been overlooked. Don't be afraid to say what you think could be wrong.

Here's an idea for you...

Make a list of questions before you see your doctor. Be prepared. It's easy to forget an important point or question, only to kick yourself when you remember on the way home.

...and another idea

Put any grievances in writing. As well as airing your complaints, spell out the help you'd like. Explain what's important to you. Writing a letter rather than collaring your counselor in the corridor means they can think about your comments and give you a more considered and constructive response.

Differences of opinion over treatment: Maybe there's been a delay in getting treatment. Or possibly you wanted a particular treatment that isn't available. These are the questions to ask:

- Why am I having this treatment?
- What are the expected benefits?
- What are the side effects?
- What will happen if I don't have this treatment?
- What are the alternatives?
- What are their expected benefits and side effects?
- Why haven't I been offered any alternatives?

Problems arising out of the doctor–patient interaction: If you feel rushed because clinics are running late, ask to come back. Comments like "I understand the clinic has run late today, so I haven't had to time to discuss everything. Could I come back soon to finish this conversation?" should get a positive response.

When you feel you haven't been taken seriously: Perhaps you've been dismissed, or made to feel like a nuisance or hysterical. If so, it's worth making a separate appointment to address those issues, rather than tacking them onto the end of a therapy session or medication review. It's a good idea to figure out what you're going to say and do a trial run with a friend beforehand. Using sentences starting with

"I" makes it more likely you'll be heard. If your sentences start with "You," there's a risk you'll end up in a cycle of accusing and blaming. Comments like: "I felt dismissed when you said, 'Stop complaining. That purple rash can't be due to the new medication,'" is more likely to lead to a meaningful discussion than, "You never listen to me. You just poison me with your chemicals."

Before you sack your psychotherapist or ditch your doctor, find out who else can help in IDEA 3, *Docs, shrinks, and quacks*.

Try another idea...

RECAP, REVIEW, REITERATE

As your conversation draws to a close, summarizing what you've understood reduces misunderstandings and keeps your conversation crisp and clear.

"So Dr. Doolittle, you're saying I can stop these pills in six months?"

"No, what I meant was, it's a good idea to continue taking them for six months after you feel completely better."

IRRECONCILABLE DIFFERENCES

Talked about your concerns and dissatisfactions but still can't see eye to eye? It's time to ask for a second opinion and agree to disagree in the meantime.

"The best doctor in the world is the veterinarian. He can't ask his patients what is the matter—he's got to just know."
WILL ROGERS, actor and humorist

Defining idea...

How did it go?

Q **Recently I read my medical notes. I was horrified. My doctor described me as "noncompliant with treatment." I felt like a naughty schoolgirl told off by the principal. I had good reasons for not slavishly following all her suggestions and am seething. How can I take things forward?**

A *"Noncompliant" is a paternalistic phrase that essentially means you have disobeyed instructions, usually to take medication. Many professionals recognize we don't always know best and try to work toward a more collaborative approach. A good first step would be writing your doctor a letter, explaining how you feel, and why you have sometimes chosen to act against her advice. Ask for an appointment to discuss your letter and explain you'd like mutual treatment decisions in the future.*

Q **I saw an arrogant smartass at the community health clinic last week. He got to me so badly that I ended up walking out of the consultation. The thing is, I need the clinic for repeat prescriptions and I go to a regular service users' group there. How can I smooth things over without apologizing for something that wasn't my fault?**

A *I don't think walking out was so terrible. More often than not, it is better to go away and cool down if you are really wound up rather than staying for an ugly scene. The way I see it, you now have two options: Either call and ask to see someone else or use some of the suggestions above to deal with Mr. Arrogant.*

39

Get off the couch

Can talking really change the way you feel? These geniuses think so. Find out what's offered and how it can help.

Psychotherapy means treatments based on talking and listening. It usually involves regular meetings at the same time, same place, for fifty minutes at least once a week, but occasionally as often as five.

FREUD SQUAD

Many psychotherapists describe their work as psychoanalytical or psychodynamic. This means they think depression has its roots in your unconscious mind or from things you've bottled up or pushed down during childhood. They treat depression by helping you become aware of these feelings and understand them. You'll often be asked to do something known as "free association." This just means saying whatever pops into your mind. These therapists use what you say to understand your unconscious mind.

Here's an idea for you...

Ask your potential psychotherapist these five questions: (1) What are your qualifications and when did you get them? (2) Which professional organizations are you accredited with? (3) What's your theoretical orientation? (4) What areas do you specialize in? (5) How much do you charge?

COUCHING YOUR PROBLEMS

Sigmund Freud, who came up with psychoanalysis, noticed when he listened to people carefully and sensitively, they developed upbeat feelings toward him. He called it transference. Later, he recognized that he also developed feelings toward his patients, sometimes optimistic, sometimes negative, and he called these feelings counter-transference. Many psychotherapists do something called "working with the transference." This means they look at the relationship and feelings between them and you and use their understanding of it to help you. Psychotherapy, and psychoanalysis in particular, traditionally had patients lying on a couch. Some still use couches, but many more provide chairs.

WHAT TO EXPECT

Use your first meeting to discover whether this type of talking treatment could be helpful. Your early sessions are usually an assessment. This means talking about the problems or worries that have brought you to therapy. Thereafter, sessions will be devoted to feelings you have about other people. This can be short-term but often takes months or years. Expect to discuss your past experiences and how these may have caused your current difficulties. Your new understanding should help you make better choices and decisions in the future.

Defining idea...

"I quit therapy because my analyst was trying to help me behind my back."
RICHARD LEWIS, comedian

FREUDIAN SLIP

Freud still has many followers, but there are therapists with a very different take. One of them was Carl Rogers. He believed we all have the capacity to find our own answers. Person-centered therapists strive to provide three so-called core conditions: empathy, congruence, and unconditional positive regard. To the rest of us, this is what they mean:

Empathy means therapists accurately understand your thoughts, feelings, and meanings and see things from your point of view.

Congruence basically means that therapists are transparent and won't hide behind theories. Instead of being false or phoney, they'll show and tell you what they think. This can be a relief, as you're not spending time second-guessing what they're really thinking about you.

Unconditional positive regard means the therapist treats you in a nonjudgmental way. You can say, think, and feel what you like without having to "earn" good vibes from your pro.

ANALYSIS PARALYSIS

Many people assume psychotherapy is always high quality and can't be harmful. I disagree and think that, like medication, it often has some unwanted effects. For instance, if your therapy goes on for years, you may become excessively dependent on therapy or your

If you like this approach but are looking for a quicker fix, cognitive analytic therapy could be right up your alley. Find out all about it in IDEA 16, *The CAT that gets the cream.*

Try another idea…

"Show me a sane man and I will cure him for you."
CARL JUNG

Defining idea…

therapist. I'm not saying that it's a bad idea to have years of therapy, but I think it is important to point out that there are risks as well as benefits. Thinking deeply about all aspects of your life can make you more anxious or miserable. You may miss a lot of work or other important activities and there are often unanticipated effects on significant relationships. It's often expensive and can become like a second mortgage.

How did it go?

Q I'm a bit confused by all these names. Could you explain the difference between a psychotherapist and a psychiatrist?

A   *A psychiatrist is a doctor with a degree in medicine and postgraduate training in detecting, diagnosing, and treating mental, emotional, and behavioral disorders. We're also able to prescribe medication. A psychotherapist is someone with specialist in-depth training in psychotherapy, including their own personal psychoanalysis. People with training and professional qualifications like psychologists, social workers, nurses, and psychiatrists are sometimes also trained in psychotherapy.*

Q I talk to my friends and family about my depression all the time and can't see how psychotherapy could help. Although I feel better for a while after unloading, talking doesn't really change anything. Or am I missing something?

A   *You may be. It's great to have supportive friends and family, but there are times when professionals can help in new ways. Psychotherapy isn't just a talking treatment. Therapists are trained to identify things you do or say that feed depression and will let you know about them in constructive and helpful ways. There might also be some things you can't tell your best friend or mother.*

40

Pedal pushers

Want a quick fix? Exercise is hard to rival. It's cheap, portable, and can make you feel better in just ten days. What are you waiting for? On your bike!

Don't like cycling? Walk away from your worries or run from your rut instead. You can do anything that leaves you gasping for breath for twenty minutes every day.

Antidepressants take two to three weeks to kick in, which is forever when you're seriously sad. So play basketball, take a Capoeira class, try Brazilian jujitsu or mountaineering. It doesn't matter what you do, as long as you get out of breath for at least twenty minutes three or more times a week. One of the best things about exercising to max your mood is instant results.

A GOOD SPORT

Exercise helps treat depression in several ways. For starters, it gets your brain's chemical communicators that are out of kilter during depression back into balance. It releases endorphins, your body's natural uplifting, depression-busting chemicals. In fact, when we exercise, our brains produce a cocktail of feel-good chemicals.

Sign up for a regular gym class, running group, or swimming night. Setting, and paying for, a routine makes it much harder to put off exercising and gives you a weekly adrenaline injection. You know it makes sense.

When you're down, just getting to the gym is a big achievement. Cut your usual workout in half and do what you can.

"People are so busy lengthening their lives with exercise they don't have time to live them."
JOHNATHAN MILLER

Scientists have found exercise's antidepressant effects could be due to a chemical that's also found in chocolate. It's called phenylethylamine and hits the same brain circuit as amphetamine, causing the so-called runner's high. Exercise also nukes a stress substance called cortisol, chilling you out. This also releases muscle tension and helps you sleep better. I don't need to tell you that poor sleep is often part of depression and messes up your quality of life. Quality sleep is a first-rate mood lifter. As if that's not enough, exercise gives us warm feelings of accomplishment, cranking up self-esteem. So what? Self-esteem is instrumental in beating depression. Most people who are depressed stop liking themselves. Getting fit, toning up, losing weight, and becoming a sexy beast should help you feel a bit better about yourself.

ON TRACK

Decided to try it? Fantastic. Whether you're exercising for the first time or coming back after a break, planning keeps you on track. Here are four tips for success:

- Choose fun exercises. Unlike school sports, this isn't about humiliation or cold showers. Unless you like that sort of thing.
- Book exercise into your planner. You know what they say, variety's the spice of life, and introducing a selection of sports into your week is more motivating than a daily date with the rowing machine.
- Why not select a team sport? You're less likely to skip out if you're letting your team down. It also helps you make friends.
- Don't give up. After three weeks it'll feel like second nature.

Made some new friends running in the park? Find out why they could be key to your recovery in IDEA 45, *I'll be there for you.*

Try another idea...

ON THE COUCH?

When depression strikes, it's tempting to curl up and sofa surf. You know you ought to get off your butt, but you can't face the gym. So here's how to stay home without staying still. Tell your cleaner to clear off and do some housework yourself. Dusting and vacuuming may seem like a unlikely antidepressant but even ironing, washing the car, or just doing dishes instead of loading the dishwasher will rev up your heartbeat. Painting the walls can be as energetic as a free weights workout. Gardening can get you out of breath quicker than a brisk walk. An hour of digging, weeding, or raking leaves may be just what the doctor ordered.

"Just do it!"
NIKE SLOGAN

Defining idea...

181

Q **Nice idea, but I can't be bothered. Can you help me get motivated?**

A *It's depression that's making you feel like this, zapping your energy and motivation. Nothing feels worth any effort. The way I see it, if you give in, you're letting depression win. Can you make yourself go for a short walk every day for a week, even just to the end of your street to mail a letter? Once you've achieved this, it'll be a cinch to build up to a longer walk on the weekend, and who knows, this time next year you could be training for a marathon.*

Q **I want to go to the gym but something always gets in the way. Any suggestions?**

A *That old chestnut. Happens to me all the time. I find it helpful to buddy up with another gym-avoider. Make exercise dates at realistic times, say, twice a week to start with, and egg each other on. Try to avoid being too virtuous in your plans. Meeting every day at 5 a.m. by the treadmill just ain't gonna happen. Exercise should be fun, so an evening's ice-skating or pole-dancing lessons may be a better bet than ten miles on the treadmill. Feeling guilty and giving yourself a hard time will make your depression worse, so if you miss a few sessions, forgive yourself and make a new start.*

41

Draw it out

Lost for words? Explore emotions, thoughts, memories, and hopes using paints, papier-mâché, clay, and collage.

Art's fun but it's also great for healing heartache. Drawing, sketching, painting, sculpting, model making, or collaging can release difficult feelings and help you cope with depression.

A PICTURE OF HEALTH

Art seems to serve a primal urge in many people. Countless psychiatric hospitals have substantial legacies of spontaneous art created over decades by patients incarcerated in asylums. Painting, drawing, or sculpting your feelings is a great way of expressing yourself when words are not enough. Pictures and models can be metaphors of distress and suffering. You don't always have to end up with a product, though. Self-expression or making a mess are valid in their own right. Art is about action, so it's great if you've being feeling out of control. And, if you choose to share your work, your point of view can be seen as well as heard.

183

Here's an idea for you... **Sculpt your recovery. Squishing clay or rolling it flat is a great way of releasing pent-up anger. You can also use clay to model and squash a person you wish you could be rid of.**

THE ART OF HEALING

Five years ago, some researchers found that a ten-week course of art therapy significantly reduced symptoms of depression in people with Alzheimer's disease. Art gave them a way of expressing things that were beyond words or even comprehension. You don't need to be Picasso to make the most of art therapy. The trick is to think of art therapy with a small *a* and capital *T*. The onus is on healing rather than award-winning pictures or objects.

PICTURE THIS

Apart from being an enjoyable and gratifying activity, art opens your eyes. When you're depressed, you often stop noticing beauty. Stopping to sketch the roses makes you aware of nice-looking things. Drawing heightens your awareness of sunsets, cityscapes, and all sorts of natural and man-made objects, deepening your curiosity and injecting some color into gray days.

Whether you're drawing a sunset, squelching and sculpting wet clay, or using your fingers to spread dollops of paint over a blank page, art is fun. Painful memories and other demons from the past are more easily dispelled in a playful environment. You don't need to buy expensive parchment paper from specialty art shops. Rolls of baking paper, newsprint, or a spare piece of wallpaper are ideal.

Defining Idea... **"Art is the stored honey of the human soul, gathered on wings of misery and travail."**
THEODORE DREISER, author

FEELING CUT UP

People with depression are often perfectionists. You, too? Making collages with images and words cut or torn from magazines and newspapers is great if your inability to draw gets you down. When you're very depressed, painting or sketching can feel like too much effort, so collages are just the thing. Why not try making a collage with a theme like loss, boredom, or the future?

Many people who like this action-oriented, creative approach also love IDEA 48, *Making a drama out of a crisis.* Art therapy works well in groups—IDEA 28, *Let them all talk,* has more on this.

Try another idea...

DRAW ON EXPERIENCE

One of the things I particularly like about this idea is that you often end up with something tangible. Many people find new meanings and metaphors in their work when returning to art produced during depression. Revisiting your work can help you recognize important undertones and nuances. Art therapists say this echoes changes in your recovery, showing you problems can be resolved. It can also provide an insight into how you feel for family and friends.

"Art opens the closets, airs out the cellars and attics. It brings healing."
JULIA CAMERON, *The Artist's Way*

Defining idea...

How did
it go?

Q   I like the sound of this but I can't draw. Everything looks different on paper than the way it does in my head. How can I improve my technique?

A   If it's any consolation, I can't draw, either. You really don't need to be a fine artist. A willingness to try a different form of self-expression is all you need. Like you, lots of people are intimidated by art therapy because it reminds them of school art lessons. Collages can be a nonthreatening way of seeing if this idea is for you, and there isn't a mark or an exam at the end.

Q   I'm thinking of seeing an art therapist but I don't really know what to expect. Any ideas?

A   Art therapists are a creative bunch and they all work slightly differently. You can see a therapist individually or in a group with other people facing difficulties. Either way, therapists provide materials for various types of artwork. Some therapists paint, others don't, as they feel it inhibits you. Some therapists make interpretations of your work, others use your product to explore feelings and events to assist recovery without imposing their idea of what your art means.

42

Settling scores

Need a pick-me-up that revives your commitment to change and boosts flagging confidence? Find out why keeping score is the answer.

If you've ever wished you were more hopeful or optimistic, then this idea will help you measure up.

COUNT ON IT

Let's say your doctor checked you for hypertension by eyeballing you and saying, "Pressure looks fine to me." Just wouldn't wash. Everyone knows you can't tell by just looking; that's why we have gadgets. One woman might tell you she's "burning up," while another says she's "lukewarm"—only a thermometer indicates whether one or both have a fever. Numbers help pros make the right diagnosis, measure symptoms and changes in their intensity or duration, and help us assess whether what we do makes any difference.

I don't know about you but I think it's lame that a straightforward "How are you feeling today?" is used to gauge despair, lost confidence, or hope. Sometimes words aren't enough to express the depth of feelings. If you feel "OK" today, but "so-so"

Here's an idea for you...

Spend an hour rating your feelings. If someone frustrates you, record your irritation on a scale of 1 to 10. Say you drop a Ming vase, rate your regret. Perhaps flowers arrive from a secret admirer, rate your surprise and happiness.

tomorrow, it's hard for friends and family to know if things are better, worse, or the same. There are times when we all need a gizmo to measure misery. This is why, in the trade, many of us use ratings to translate words into numbers.

MARKS OUT OF TEN

Let's say you rated how you were feeling on a scale of 1 to 10 where 10 was the best you'd ever felt and 1 the worst. I asked John, a forty-year-old portrait painter, the same question. He put his mood at 3/10. Here's what happened next:

Me: Why not 1/10?
John: Well, some things are still going OK. I'm getting along well with Lynne and she helps me out.
Me: Maybe it'll help to think about the closest to 10/10 your mood's ever been.
John: Four years ago it would've been 9/10. I'd just been promoted, met Lynne, and started playing golf. Everything was going right.
Me: Were there things you were doing differently then?

Defining idea...

"I measure every grief I meet
With analytic eyes;
I wonder if it weighs like mine,
Or has an easier size."
EMILY DICKINSON

John: Yeah, I was making more effort, you know, with how I look, shaving and stuff like that. I was seeing my friends more, playing golf and inviting them over.

Me: What might you need to do to get closer to 4/10?

John: I could force myself to get out a bit more, maybe have a dinner party.

Me: Say you did those things, what do you think you'd notice was different about yourself?

John: I probably wouldn't feel so fed up all the time.

Me: Do you think Lynne would notice anything different?

John: (laughing) She'd probably be relieved I wasn't moping around the house.

How will your friends and family treat you differently when your mood moves from 4/10 to 8/10? Using questions like this can make miracles happen. Prepare to be amazed in IDEA 11, *Nothing short of a miracle.*

Try another idea...

WHAT'S THE SCORE?

Can you see how keeping score makes John more aware of how he's feeling, shows him what he's already doing that helps, and what more he needs to do? Great. Over to you. How motivated do you feel to try this idea? Let's say you're moderately enthused at 5/10. What would it take to move one point from 5 to 6? Not sure? Let me put it another way. When you move from 5 to 6, what will you be doing that you're not doing now? When you move from 5 to 6, what would I notice was different about you? As you think through steps you can take to move up the scale, you'll discover what needs to be done to bring about even more changes. Got the hang of it? Fantastic. Once you start keeping score, you'll realize you can use numbers in almost every part of your life. The applications are endless.

If you find it hard to pick a number off an imaginary scale in your head, why not draw scales like the ones in this Idea and circle your answers? Might look like a lot of work, but once you've decided which scores you'll keep, it's easy to make a tally sheet and photocopy enough for a couple of weeks.

Mood

1	2	3	4	5	6	7	8	9	10

I feel lower than a worm

I'm the happiest I've ever felt

Confidence

1	2	3	4	5	6	7	8	9	10

I feel like hiding in the corner

I could stand up and give a talk to 1,000 people

Self-esteem

1	2	3	4	5	6	7	8	9	10

I feel like a worthless piece of scum

I'm on top of the world

How much I feel like changing

1   2   3   4   5   6   7   8   9   10

I can't be
bothered to
do anything

I want a
big-time life
makeover

Hope for the future

1   2   3   4   5   6   7   8   9   10

I can't
believe
anything will
get better

I'm very
hopeful life
will be better

How did it go?

Q   My mood changes quickly. How can I put a number on my feelings?

A   *Imagine ratings as snapshots. If you specify a time limit, ratings become much more useful. They become equivalent to those before-and-after photographs you see on makeover shows. Like today, I feel 5/10 compared to yesterday, when I only felt 2/10. Or last year was 6/10 overall but this year is 7/10.*

Q   Numbers leave me cold. Saying "I feel 6/10" sounds artificial. Any tips?

A   *I agree it's a bit fake. The trouble is that although "pissed off" expresses how you feel, there's little way of knowing how and why your feelings change from day to day. Keeping score doesn't just give you a way of measuring change, it helps exploit this to hasten your recovery.*

43

All hands on deck

If you've had one of those days when you just can't take any more, this hands-on idea is a fail-safe route to getting your va-va-voom back.

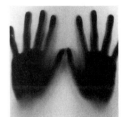

Having a languorous massage is an excellent way to improve your quality of life, helping you live with debilitating symptoms.

Forget those lewd connotations. The sort of massage I'm talking about is soothing, simple, and sensuous. A way of caressing, pressing, and kneading your body, relieving tension and reducing pain, preferably by a trained massage therapist. It leaves you feeling calm and cared for.

REACH OUT AND TOUCH

Being touched sensitively by another human being makes us feel warm and fuzzy. If we're deprived of touch, we often feel lonely and uneasy. Massage produces chemical changes in the brain and lowers levels of stress hormones. Teenage moms who received massage therapy compared to those having relaxation therapy were less depressed and less anxious both by their own accounts and based on professional observations. A study at the University of South Carolina found that women who lost a child were found to be less depressed after receiving therapeutic massage.

Here's an idea for you...

Give acupuncture a try—some forms of depression seem to respond well to this treatment. Perhaps your doctor can recommend a local needle wizard.

Under pressure? Here are just some of the ways massage can help:

- Reduces stress and tension
- Relieves pain
- Increases levels of serotonin, protecting against depression
- Increases endorphins, the body's natural painkillers
- Strengthens the immune system

RUBBED THE WRONG WAY?

Scientists at the Touch Research Institute in Florida verified that massage plays a role in reducing stress. They split fifty people into two groups. One group had a chair massage twice a week for five weeks while the others were asked to relax in a chair at the same times. At the end of five weeks, both groups were less depressed, but the group who'd been massaged was less stressed.

Defining idea...

"Years ago massage was a big part of nursing. There was so much care, so much touch, so much goodness conveyed through massage."
DR. JOAN BORYSENKO, medical scientist and psychologist

STROKES OF GENIUS

So you want to go for a massage but are confused by all the different names? Aromatherapy massage uses oils applied in long, flowing strokes, called "effleurage." These oils can be soothing or invigorating. Swedish massage is much more energetic. It's intended to energize by stimulating your circulation. Feldenkrais, Rolfing, and Hellerwork are varieties of deep-tissue massage, which are great for taking strain out of deeper muscles and can help with injuries.

A HEAD START

Tension headache? Massage your forehead and feel stress melting away. First, cozy up in a comfortable chair. Now put the fingertips of your right hand on your right eyebrow. Pressing quite hard, slide your fingertips along your eyebrow until you reach your temple. Massage your temple by making small circles with your fingertips. Finally, repeat using your left hand on your left eyebrow. If you can, spend a few minutes sitting quietly with your eyes closed.

Feeling too fat to face the masseuse? Hitting the gym can get both your body and mind back into great shape, so make **IDEA 40, Pedal pushers**, your next stop.

Try another idea...

DO IT YOURSELF

Obviously it's a little tricky to massage yourself in those hard to reach places where tension builds up, so why not buddy up with a friend? Giving each other a neck and shoulder massage saves you the embarrassment of stripping. You can do this with a work colleague and without leaving your desk. Just six steps can take you from feeling frazzled and fed-up to light as a feather. Here's how:

1. Support your friend's head in your left hand and turn it gently toward the right. Move your right hand to make a firm stroking movement out from the middle of her back to the top of her arm.
2. Now move back along the top of her shoulder, then up the back of her neck to the bottom of her head.
3. Make small circles along the back of her neck.
4. Next, make some gentle strokes across the top of her shoulder.

"In the absence of touching and being touched, people of all ages can sicken and grow touch starved."
DIANE ACKERMAN, *A Natural History of the Senses*

Defining idea...

5. Tilt her head back to the middle using both your hands to support her head under her neck.
6. Now support her head with your right hand and turn it to the left, repeating these steps for the other side and finish by making some more circles on the back of her neck.

How did *it go?*

Q **I've had postpartum depression twice and am now pregnant again. My friend says baby massage prevents postpartum depression. Is she right?**

A *While it's true that research has suggested baby massage helps mothers with postpartum depression bond better with their babies, there's no scientific proof to back up your friend's claim. Lots of moms find it relaxing, though, and feel happier afterward. If you want to give it a try, your pediatrician will be able to put you in touch with local classes.*

Q **I don't feel comfortable with the idea of being touched all over by a stranger, but wouldn't mind someone "doing" my feet. Do you think reflexology might help me?**

A *Qualified massage therapists are used to people feeling nervous and will cover you with drapes and towels, so don't worry about lying there on display. Many people swear by reflexology, an ancient type of foot massage. There's no evidence that it improves symptoms of depression, but I figure if it helps you put your best foot forward, go for it. Indian head massage or just a head and neck job will also spare your blushes.*

Sexual healing

Feeling blue? Lost that loving feeling? Find your lost libido and arouse a bit of joy.

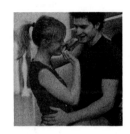

Lots of people with depression lose interest in sex. Discover how to perk up your passions and your mood.

If you're looking for some really personal therapy, good sex is a lovely remedy. When you make love, your body releases natural feel-good chemicals called endorphins. They give you a euphoric buzz, lift your mood, increase pleasure, and reduce pain. When you orgasm, your body releases a hormone called oxytocin that makes you feel loved up and blissful. All very well, but what if you're just not in the mood? First, you're not alone. One in five people have low or lost libido at any one time.

SEX AND DRUGS

Certain antidepressants can cause your lowered sex drive to plummet to new depths. Selective serotonin reuptake inhibitors (SSRIs) are the most common culprits. One of their side effects is zapping brains of one of our major sexual pleasure chemicals, called dopamine. Ditching drugs is rarely your best strategy, but there are things you can do to reclaim your lust.

Here's an idea for you...

To get into a sensual mood, lie back and relax in a warm bath before going to bed. Unwind and imagine tensions and strains washing away. Pamper yourself with soothing bath lotions and sweet-smelling massage oils. If you treat yourself like an Adonis or Aphrodite goddess, you'll feel like one.

KISS IT BETTER

If your sex drive has driven off, rebuild your relationship by kissing and cuddling. When did you last have a really good make out session? Set aside at least ten minutes and snuggle. Hug, rub your lips together, make your partner smile, and enjoy new and forgotten sensations.

IT'S A DATE

Some sexperts suggest booking lovemaking times into your schedules, just as you'd book meetings. It might sound unromantic, but it can get you back into it. Avoid putting off sex because you haven't got time for a three-hour love-in. A quickie is better than nothing and the more sex you have, the more you'll feel like having.

...and another idea

Serve up some oysters. They're rich in zinc, a trace element essential for healthy sex organs. Caviar or mussels do the trick, too.

BOOKS AT BEDTIME

I'm sure you've heard it said that your biggest sexual organ is your brain. So liberate your libido by investigating some "adult" literature. It's generally accepted that men get turned on by pictures and women by words, but hey, who says we have to conform to gender stereotypes? Bear in mind your understated erotica might be your partner's intolerable hard-core pornography.

RAUNCH PAD

Rev up your yearnings by making romance a top priority. You don't need a book to tell you that binge drinking and smoking lots of cannabis are bad news for your moods and your love life. So spoil yourself instead with sensual pleasures like silk pajamas or a fur throw for your bed. Jilt the gym and have a bedroom workout instead. Treat yourself and your partner to a candlelit dinner, slow dancing, a romantic film—corny clichés, maybe, but they work. So does getting close and personal on a rug in front of an open fire. If you've only got a radiator, swapping the glow of the TV for a candlelit bedroom helps, too.

As any new mom or shift worker knows, sleep deprivation plays havoc with your sex drive. Get the right balance of bedroom activities by following the tips in IDEA 8, *Counting sheep.*

Try another idea...

BETWEEN THE SHEETS

Remember the good feelings you had after making love? Rekindle those vibes. Swap your polyester bedsheets for silk or satin ones and re-create your old memories or try out some new fantasies.

Skipping sex because you're too tired diminishes your interest even more. Sex can be fantastically soporific, making you more likely to get a good night's uninterrupted shut-eye.

Arlene: "You're crazy!"
Phil: "That's right! Not having sex for twelve years will do that to a person!"
CITY SLICKERS

Defining idea...

How did
it go?

Q **I'm single and too depressed to start a new relationship. From time to time I've ended up having a one-night stand or brief fling, but it's never made me feel any better. Where am I going wrong?**

A *Emotional intimacy is an important part of the health benefits of sex. One-night stands can work against you, worsening your depression by making you anxious or worried about diseases, guilty about having broken your own values, or just feeling used and empty.*

Q **I've got some problems at work—my boss is really down on me—and I just can't think of anything else at the moment. What should I do?**

A *According to Dr. Ava Cadell, a sexologist, "When you're upset about something it can be so overwhelming that your entire focus is on the problem, and the last thing you want to do is to have sex, even though it would be the best thing you could do. Sex can actually clear the mind and help you come up with some good solutions."*

Q **My other half says he read in a men's magazine that semen is a natural antidepressant. Is this true?**

A *Nice try, but I wouldn't swallow his theory. I'm afraid there's no proof to substantiate his claim.*

45

I'll be there for you

Are hugs the new drugs? Isolation worsens depression, but good friends can raise low moods. Discover the restorative powers of confiding relationships.

A chat over coffee with a friend could help your depression as much as pills or therapy.

Medical students and trainee psychiatrists learn by rote the classic Camberwell Study, but I'm often surprised how few people with depression have heard of it. In the 1970s, sociologist and all-around nice guy George Brown paired up with psychiatrist Tirril Harris and interviewed over a thousand women in Camberwell (a poor part of London). They found women without good, caring, intimate friendships were more likely to get depressed. There's no reason to think this doesn't apply to guys, too. The bottom line? Friendships are the single most effective safeguard against depression.

CAFÉ CULTURE

Tirril Harris carried on her groundbreaking work. Twenty years later, she studied another group of depressed women. They were randomly assigned to two groups. One group met a befriender, the other was placed on a waiting list for one.

Here's an idea for you... **If you're fed up with your friends, become a volunteer in your neighborhood and make new ones. No matter if it's a soup run for local homeless people, first aid at football matches, or a prison writing project, volunteering is a good way of combating depression and forging friendships.**

Befrienders were volunteers acting as compassionate sounding boards. They often met for chats over coffee. Guess what? Nearly three-quarters of women with befrienders recovered from depression compared to only 45 percent of those on the waiting list. Remarkably, that's about the same success rate as drugs or therapy.

PEOPLE NEED PEOPLE

Even when you feel like staying home alone, remind yourself that seeing more of your friends lifts your mood. Just knowing someone cares about you can help. Confiding in close pals helps you think through why you're down. Good friends are usually great listeners and able to suggest solutions you hadn't thought of.

Defining idea... *"Friends are God's apology for relatives."*
HUGH KINGSMILL, British poet

Defining idea... *"In addition to my other numerous acquaintances, I have one more intimate confidant. My depression is the most faithful mistress I have known—no wonder, then, that I return the love."*
SOREN KIERKEGAARD

Is your depression making you think you don't deserve friends? When you're down, being in company is almost always better than being alone. Although you might not feel like going out, try to stay in touch with friends. If the phone seems daunting, why not email, text, or send postcards?

GET A GRIP

Some friends mean well but say useless things like, "All you need is a new boyfriend." Comments like this aren't usually malicious, so try filtering out bad advice and let your friends know telling you to snap out of it or pull yourself together makes things worse. Friends don't often know how to help. You might need to spell it out by saying things like "Listen to me without judging what I say" or "When you go out, invite me."

Sometimes only someone who's been through the same stuff will *really* understand what you're going through. To find out more about self-help groups and group therapy, check out IDEA 28, *Let them all talk.*

Try another idea...

How did it go?

Q **I try to talk to my partner about how bad I'm feeling but he seems to switch off and isn't very helpful. I feel lonely and it's as if he's just not interested in me when I'm depressed. I hate being a burden on him, but really need more understanding. Should I leave him?**

A *This is a common problem. Big "should I stay or should I go?" decisions are best left for when you're feeling better. When we're depressed, everything seems dark and hopeless. Your partner might be a useless loser, or a decent guy who doesn't know how to help. Sometimes partners are too close or even part of the problem. When this happens, they're not best placed to help you out of your depression. Sometimes when people are depressed,* *we're not a bundle of laughs. I'm not saying you're like this, but when you're with a depressed person 24/7 they can sometimes seem unreasonable or even pathetic. Rather than tear your hair out in frustration over your man's lack of compassion, I suggest you find another close friend. Tell her how you feel and let her know what she can do to help.*

Q My friends have made me depressed by taking advantage of me. I'm the only one who's still single and they're always treating me as an unpaid babysitter and using my spare room to accommodate visiting in-laws. They're partly to blame for how bad I'm feeling but they just can't see it. How can I get them to realize?

A You're not going to like this but you have two options: waste time and energy trying to get your friends to see it from your point of view or start looking after yourself better. Your friends can't force you to babysit or take in their unwanted relatives. It might sound harsh but they're putting this on you because they can get away with it. You can turn this around by choosing to say no. Not allowing people to take advantage is one of the toughest challenges I've overcome. Now I'm rarely taken for granted and my efforts are appreciated. I'm much happier.

46

Imagine

Yearning for a calming, captivating technique to soothe your soul? Find out how visualization can relax and revive you.

Visualization means using your mind to create pictures. Use it to relax, fall asleep, or get back in the party mood.

Creating pictures or scenes in your mind's eye is a great way to relax, but can be used in other ways as well. Visualization helped women suffering from postpartum depression. Researchers observed women who had given birth to their first child for the first four weeks following the births. Women who took part in visualization techniques had reduced depression and anxiety but also improved self-esteem compared to women who didn't.

Have you ever thought, "What's the point? I'll mess it up anyway so why bother?" Instead of predicting how things are going to end up, why not visualize them the way you'd like them? Some people visualize their antidepressants as a waterfall, washing away depression. Or you can liven up by imagining yourself doing something you enjoy.

Here's an idea for you...

Make a list of all the possible solutions to your deep-rooted problems and imagine each solution is written on a door. Now imagine yourself going through each door in turn. What do you find on the other side? If it's not what you'd like, cross back over the threshold and go through a different door.

GETTING STARTED

If you want to try it, the best way to start is using visualization techniques to relax. If you're feeling stressed, here's how it can help.

Find a quiet place where you won't be disturbed. Close your eyes for a few minutes. Cast your mind back to the time in your life you felt most deeply relaxed. Some people like to think of a vacation, but feel free to choose anywhere. Imagine yourself in that calm place now. Try to bring it to life vividly, using all your senses. What can you see? What can you hear? What can you taste? What can you smell? What can you feel? Stay in that place as long as it takes to feel calm. It needs practice, but once you can picture your calming place, you've got an individualized, portable stress-buster.

A BRAIN OF TWO HALVES

Creating pictures in your mind's eye can help you achieve things you never thought possible. Nobody's really sure how this works, but one idea is that visualization stimulates the right half of your brain—that's the part dealing with emotions and creativity. In most people, the left half is responsible for reasoning, verbal ability, and making logical conclusions. Stimulating the right half balances out the left, leaving you more relaxed and able to see things in a quirkier way.

TESTING TIMES

Terrified of exams? I used to convince myself that I'd fail. And guess what? I did fail a fair few and think I underperformed in many more. It really got me down. I've since learned there's

Having problems imagining or envisaging? Visualization can be difficult if you're feeling panicky. Check out IDEA 23, *Don't panic*.

Try another idea...

no surer route to failure than predicting it. Spending five minutes a day during revision periods visualizing the exam room helped enormously. I imagined opening the paper and being pleased to see I could answer each question easily. Top athletes use visualization during the last stages of training. A similar technique works for interviews, too.

MAKE IT WORK

No success at job interviews? Visualization helps you make a great first impression and maximize your performance. Fears about rejection can make you overcautious, underconfident, and look defeated before you've even started. I'd encourage you to imagine your wildest dreams coming true. Visualize wowing the panel with your answers, exceling at presentations, speaking fluently and articulately, and then being offered the job. Enjoy it. How does it feel? Of course, no one can promise it will go like that on the day of, but mental dress rehearsals will help you give your best performance. Cultivating optimism and enthusiasm will positively affect interviewers' responses to you and, if you're not offered the job this time, it'll help you bounce back rather than sinking into desolation.

"It is never too late to be what you might have been."
GEORGE ELIOT

Defining idea...

How did it go?

Q **I struggle to actually see anything in my mind's eye. How can I get better at it?**

A *Lots of people struggle to create scenes in their mind. Practicing when you're calm helps you get the hang of it, so you can use it easily when you really need it. You might be one of those people who only thinks in words and never in pictures. If this is the case, use your own wordscapes to imagine that dream outcome.*

Q **Isn't raising hopes only going to deepen my depression when what i'm trying for doesn't materialize?**

A *Probably not. The fear of failure is, in my book, the biggest depressant of them all. As a rule, contented people generally don't worry about failures, regarding them as setbacks and part of a learning experience.*

47

Because you're worth it

Feeling down in the dumps with nothing to look forward to? In need of something to put a smile on your face? Some self-indulgent me time always helps.

If your get up and go has got up and gone, this idea will give you the strength to go after it.

Feeling the worse for wear? A little pampering and preening can be incredibly revitalizing, raising your mood, confidence, and self-esteem.

RISE AND SHINE

Waking up early and can't get back to sleep? Instead of lying there worrying, injecting a little effort into your morning routine will bring daylong benefits. Looking chic and sophisticated compared to dull and dreary makes a whopping difference to how people treat you and how you feel. Not convinced? How would you feel in response to these two statements?

"You look really tired. Are you OK?"
"Wow, you look amazing. Love the new suit."

Here's an
idea for
you...

**Perk yourself up with a
pedicure. Relaxing foot
massages can nurture, cleanse,
energize, and relax your body
and mind.**

It might sound obvious but wearing vibrant colors will give you more zip and zing than dressing in drab browns or grays.

If you're strapped for cash right now, then perhaps it's time to check out some secondhand shops. You should be able to inject some pizzazz into your wardrobe on the cheap (and a fashion mistake that hasn't crippled your credit card is much easier to live with!). If the secondhand pickings are slim where you live, then give eBay a whirl. There are lots of interesting clothes to be had out there in cyberspace.

MAKE UP YOUR MIND

Putting on makeup might be the last thing you feel like doing when you're depressed, but the old saying "outer beauty, inner strength" has a lot of truth in it. Ever wondered why your granny called it war paint? Researchers investigated the effects of makeup on our moods by giving daily makeovers to elderly people suffering from incontinence. Three months into the experiment, a third of the elderly were out of their incontinence pads. Makeup helped them recover their dignity and sense of worth.

Defining
idea...

*"I'm tired of all this nonsense
about beauty being only skin-
deep. That's deep enough.
What do you want, an
adorable pancreas?"*
JEAN KERR, writer and lyricist

Many hospitals employ beauticians to improve the well-being of cancer patients. Most psychiatric departments are sadly lagging behind. I once worked on a ward where one of the nurses ran a weekly "beauty group." She styled people's hair, did mini manicures, and generally made people look and feel like a million dollars. It convinced me that the trusty lipstick and mascara combo can transform the way you feel. Treating yourself to some new vibrant eye colors might seem like just an instant pick-me-up, but it also gives you a little confidence boost every time you use them.

Blissed out? You will be after discovering the mood-boosting benefits of massage in IDEA 43, *All hands on deck.*

Try another idea...

HAIR'S AN IDEA FOR YOU

Are perms the new Prozac? Probably not, but if you're fed up or feeling frumpy, half an hour at your hairdresser is great for hauling up your humor. Many hairdressers have first-rate listening skills. Mine's certainly got the sort of interested empathy many shrinks can only dream of, and a humble cut and blow-dry can turn into an impromptu therapy session. His enthusiasm and bonhomie are remarkably infectious and I've lost count of the times I've gone in dejected, looking disheveled, and come out sleek, sexy, and smiling. The lift you get might not last longer than your retouched roots, but it could become the highlight of your month.

LOOK GOOD, FEEL GREAT

Tense and on edge? Unwind and rejuvenate at a beauty parlor or day spa. While a Brazilian bikini wax may well make you cry, a hot stone massage, age-defying facial, or airbrush tan are sure to make you feel like one of the happy people. Guys, no need to be shy. Take your pick from wet shaves, sports massage, and other indulgences from the male spruce-up menu.

"Happiness begins when one decides not to be something, but to be someone."
COCO CHANEL

Defining idea...

Q **All this coddling just isn't me. I had my hair cut but still feel sad inside. How can I find happiness in a tube of lipstick?**

A *Ever heard the phrase "fake it till you make it"? A makeover can help you make-believe that you're a secure, happy person. All of us are affected by the way other people respond to us. If the vibe you give off is "I'm down and I couldn't care less about myself," people will pick up on that and treat you differently.*

Q **As a poor student, I'm not able to afford spa weekends or designer clothes. What can I do?**

A *Indulging yourself doesn't have to mean spending like a football pro's wife. Lots of perfect pick-me-ups come with modest price tags: traditional sandalwood shaving soap, lavender-scented bath oil, nail polish. Good hairdressers are often looking for models (read: freebie hairdo) and beauty therapy schools frequently offer half-price treatments with their students. Keep a lookout, too, for warehouse sales and designer sample events.*

48

Making a drama out of a crisis

Discover a dramatic solution for your depression. Stop being a mere spectator in life's tragicomedy and get back in the director's chair. Discover how to set the scene for recuperation and stage your recovery.

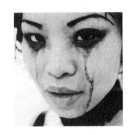

Doing drama doesn't mean you have to build a theater in your yard or erect a stage in your spare room. To the ancient Greeks, drama simply meant something that is acted out or lived through.

ACTING OUT

Both psychodrama and drama therapy explore feelings using actions. They usually involve group work, although you can do drama therapy one on one. Psychodrama was developed by Jacob Levy Moreno, a Viennese doctor who came up with the idea after watching children playing in a park. In psychodrama, a supportive and encouraging group enacts ordeals from the past, current difficulties, and future challenges. Drama therapy uses improvization, mimes, mask making, rituals, role-

Here's an idea for you...

Join a local drama group. Taking part in an amateur dramatics production will develop your spontaneity, resourcefulness, and self-expression. You'll gain confidence and playing different parts can help change self-defeating patterns.

playing, dance, storytelling, play writing, puppetry, and theater games to explore personal and interpersonal stuff. It can also help you develop poise, self-confidence, and alternative approaches to deal with difficulties.

FUN AND GAMES

Theater games give you a chance to try out exercises actors use to delve deeper into characters. These playful approaches are a brilliant way of seeing difficult circumstances from others' points of view.

MIME

If you've ever seen an old Charlie Chaplin film, you'll know how much emotion can be conveyed without words. Mime can be valuable therapy if you're shy or awkward with words. How would you mime what depression feels like?

Defining idea...

"All the world's a stage,
And all the men and women merely players;
They have their exits and their entrances;
And one man in his time plays many parts,
His acts being seven ages."
WILLIAM SHAKESPEARE, *As You Like It*

BEHIND THE MASK

I make masks as a way of confronting and facing difficult emotions. Creating masks out of plaster, paper, leather, and fabric helps you capture a state of mind, feeling, or daydream. You might want to use them as part of acting out scenarios, but many people find the process of creating them beneficial, opening doors to better expression and communication.

WHO'S BEEN SITTING IN MY CHAIR?

The so-called empty chair technique was developed by Gestalt guru Frederick Perls. This is how it goes. Sit facing an empty chair, and in your mind's eye, sit someone there who has given you grief, anyone you like, dead or alive. You might find putting a photo of them there helps. Next tell them things you wish you'd been able to say, but never had the chance. Say whatever you need to: shout, cry, rant, blame, accuse. Swapping seats and hearing your views from the other perspective can be enlightening and helpful.

STALEMATE

You'll need to get together a team for this. Everyone comes up with a real life predicament and writes it on an index card. Put all the index cards in a shoe box and pick one out. Next, each person acts out their responses, actions, or reactions to the dilemma.

SERIOUS PLAYTIME

Role-plays are great because they give you a chance to rehearse and practice your responses to difficult situations. Unlike real life, you're free to try, fail, and try again until you succeed.

I used to get stressed out before clinical exams. Then I started role-playing with colleagues. We did a lot of "dummy runs," taking turns playing candidates and

*Depression and anxiety often go hand in hand. IDEA 23, **Don't panic**, gives you strategies to manage panic attacks, free-floating anxiety, and all those irrational fears.*

Try another idea...

"When I read great literature, great drama, speeches, or sermons, I feel that the human mind has not achieved anything greater than the ability to share feelings and thoughts through language."
JAMES EARL JONES, actor

Defining idea...

215

examiners. This didn't banish all my exam nerves but it made them bearable and helped me give a winning performance on the day of the exam.

Fooling around by role-playing a person you admire can be helpful if your confidence is low. Taking on some of their attributes, if only for half an hour, helps you emulate your mentors and give depression the boot.

How did it go?

Q **I've read a bit about psychodrama and was confused by all the stuff on "auxiliary egos." Could you explain what that's about?**

A   *In psychodrama, there are a few new names to get used to. There's a protagonist, the person who chooses an event from her life and provides enough information for it to be enacted; auxiliary egos are other patients or group members who act out other people from the protagonist's life; an audience made up of other group members who observe and respond to the drama; and the therapist, who is known as the director. I wouldn't worry too much about this though. You'll quickly get the hang of it if you try it. Nobody will force you to be a protagonist unless you want to. Being part of the audience is a good start.*

Q **I'd like to try this but I'm not a very good actor. Does that matter?**

A   *Not at all. You can learn to change unhelpful behaviors, try new life skills, express difficult feelings, and learn to solve problems without any Oscar-winning performances.*

49

Shades of gray

Depressed people tend to think in all-or-nothing terms. There's never been a better time to find out why gray's the new black and white.

If you're not the "life and soul of the party," you must be "dull as dishwater." Job not perfect? It must be a nightmare. Son not top of the class? He must be backward. Does self-imposed perfectionism mean you never measure up?

Most things aren't major disasters or cause for great celebration. Life tends to throw us a mixture of pain and pleasure. When you're depressed, you can easily lose perspective on this, as depression often makes us think in all-or-nothing terms. When I was at school, I used to think if I didn't get straight As, it meant I was a failure. If I didn't get an A, it felt as bad as if I had failed. One of my patients ran the London marathon. Because he didn't come in first in his running club, he felt there had been no point in taking part.

Here's an
idea for
you... **Start keeping track of times
you use the words "always,"
"never," "completely," or
"typical." Get into the habit of
asking yourself if you could be
exaggerating. Perhaps you're
only focusing on things that
have gone wrong and forgetting
all the stuff you've achieved.
Could you be so absorbed in
your weaknesses that you
forget your strengths? Are you
assuming you can't do anything
to change things? Isn't it time
to stop losing sleep over the
way things used to be? Instead,
focus on how they are now.**

BLACK AND WHITE MAKES YOU BLUE

Experts call this "black-and-white thinking."
And far from just being a sign of depression, it
worsens it, dragging you lower and lower.
Black-and-white thinking makes you feel more
depressed, worried, stressed, or angry. It also
stops you from doing things that'd help you
feel better, like seeing friends.

GRAY DAYS

Seeing the world without shades of gray is a
primitive form of self-protection. For example,
if there's a fire, you're more likely to survive if
you make a snap decision to get out than if
you hang around weighing the pros and cons
of various exit routes. So it's great for life-threatening crises, but not so hip or hot
for everyday stuff. In fact, it has some serious limitations. When you use black-and-
white thinking in non-emergencies, you sink deeper into depression. The more
your thoughts are polarized into extremes, the more your moods will swing like a
chimpanzee at feeding time. You'll start having all-or-nothing thoughts like "Our
vacation was a complete disaster," "Nothing ever works out for me," "My wife's
always so selfish," "My sister's got the perfect house but mine is just a hovel." Very
few relationships, homes, jobs, or friendships are worthy of such a total write-off,
but have good and bad elements in them.

MIND YOUR LANGUAGE

Never happy? Always let down by others? Completely inadequate? Nothing to look forward to? Always do your best to fight depression? Completely ineffectual? Never good enough? Always going to be like this? Typical—everything always goes wrong. If any of these phrases sound familiar, you've become a victim of the black-and-white thoughts squad. Recognizing this is happening is a major step, as it helps you move on.

Like anything new, moving from all or nothing to shades of gray can be hard. If you've been swinging back and forth between two extremes, it can be difficult to believe in options, compromise, or middle ground. Think back to the last time you used black-and-white thinking. When did one of these phrases last pass your lips?

- Nothing helps.
- I'll never feel better.
- It'll be terrible.
- What's the point in trying?
- I've got to get it completely right.

What thoughts went through your mind? How did you feel afterward? Did you notice any aches or pains, anxiety, or sick feelings? You can't always control how you feel, but you can control these all-or-nothing thoughts.

Keeping a daily log is a great way to keep tabs on black-and-white thinking and encourage yourself to introduce those all important gray hues. IDEA 4, *Dear diary*, helps you put it write.

Try another idea...

"Life is not a spelling bee where one mistake wipes out all the things we have done right."
RABBI HAROLD S. KUSHNER

Defining idea...

How did it go?

Q **After being terribly depressed for three years, I tried giving up black-and-white thinking and it helped me become more levelheaded. I was starting to feel better, when suddenly, a couple of weeks ago, it all went wrong. I'm back where I started and I can't see myself getting any better. What's the point?**

A *I don't doubt that you feel worse than you did a few weeks ago, but are you really back where you started? My guess is you're feeling bitterly disappointed at the stark contrast between how you feel now and how you felt when things seemed to be getting better. See this as a setback, no more, no less. If you're able to try out some new gray thinking, great, but if you don't feel up to it right now, don't worry. Feeling hopeless and wondering what the point is, is unfortunately part of depression, but it doesn't mean it's how things really are.*

Q **I'm worried this way of thinking will rob me of the few certainties I hang on to. How will I cope?**

A *Sorry to break it to you, but there are no certainties.*

50

Get me out of here

Do vacations leave you feeling stressed, tired, broke, and more depressed than when you left home? Not anymore. Use this travel guide to get to new heights.

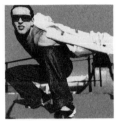

These inspired solutions will help you jet off on a vacation that will re-energize you, rather than leaving your nerves as raw and frazzled as your sunburnt nose.

EASY DOES IT

For a vacation that's all healing and no stress, the trick is planning around the three Rs:

- Relaxation
- Recreation
- Recuperation

An ideal start is finding a vacation destination where the pace of life is slower than what you're used to. There's a good chance you'll return re-energized, overflowing with enthusiasm, and ready to win your fight against depression. Of course, a little bit of activity is good, but the balance should be more comforting beachfront spa or

Here's an idea for you...

Try to make your good vacation mood last longer than your tan. Did you enjoy a dip in the ocean? Then try to go to your local pool a couple of times a week. Close your eyes and pretend you're back in the Caribbean for a few minutes.

cheeringly luxe après-ski rather than advanced desert quad biking or championship snowboarding.

BE PREPARED

Unrealistic expectations are a top reason for holiday stress. A last-minute discount break might look too good to miss, but many depressed people find sudden changes in their plans or environment too much. Let's face it, there's no point saving on a last-minute trip to Zimbabwe if the stress and upheaval triples your therapy bill in the long run. Planning vacations in advance, savoring small details, and knowing where you're going to stay will help ease you into a new routine and make sure you get the most out of it. It's worth taking time to learn about the country or town you're visiting, getting an overview of its history, culture, and must-sees.

Defining idea...

"Twenty years from now you will be more disappointed by the things you didn't do than by the ones you did. So throw off the bowlines. Sail away from the safe harbor. Catch the trade winds in your sails. Explore. Dream. Discover."
MARK TWAIN

Making arrangements to go away, booking tickets, and negotiating busy stations or airports are all inherently stressful and harder to do when you're feeling depressed. Now's the time to call on friends who have asked what they can do to help. Delegate and prioritize. If you can, take a few days' leave before your journey. Getting organized means you'll be able to chill for a few days before you travel, zoning out of your normal routine slowly rather than with a jolt. Planning a treat for when you get home will give you something to look forward to during your trip home, rather than just dreading a deluge of emails or bills. Finishing housework before you go means you won't have to come home and start cleaning.

Even if you're away with friends or on a family vacation, building a bit of "me time" into your break can make a massive difference to your mood. Find out why in IDEA 47, *Because you're worth it*.

Try another idea...

FLIGHTS OF FANCY

Seeking out some far-flung friends might seem like a good idea, but the emotional demands of reunions, combined with the stresses involved in being a good houseguest, are a recipe for misery. My brother-in-law Tim loves quoting the old Chinese proverb, "Fish and guests go bad after two days," but he's right and chances are you'll pick up the "Why did we invite you?" vibe. By all means, drop in on old friends, but reconnecting with your urge to splurge and staying in a hotel or guesthouse will go a long way toward ensuring a happy vacation.

Q   **Going on vacation never fails to cheer me up. The problem starts when I get back. I feel so down, my husband thinks it isn't worth going away in the first place. Do you have any suggestions for coping with these homecoming depressions?**

How did it go?

A   *I know the feeling. You come home, the washing machine's flooded, there are a thousand emails in your inbox, and you can't open the door for piled-up bills. Don't despair. There are things you can do to avoid post-vacation blues and keep your feel-good glow. Try to bring some of your holiday good mood home with you. Try to find some of the food you enjoyed on your break. Only do things that are really important. I usually come back to lots of apparently urgent messages, but it's surprising how many of them can actually wait a day or two. It's also too easy to fall into the trap of working extra hard to make up for the time you were away. Be firm with yourself and make a run for it at quitting time.*

Q   I enjoy going away and find it gives me a much-needed boost. Unfortunately, jet lag makes me tired and disoriented, wrecking the first few days of my break. I'm doing all the sensible things, like resetting my watch to local time and taking a nap when I arrive. What else can I do?

A   Resetting your watch is a great idea, but I'm not so sure about taking a nap. It might sound counterintuitive to stay awake, but I'm afraid napping can play havoc with your body clock, leaving you more out of sync and miserable. Instead, try getting out. Spending time in sunlight is a great way to reset your body's natural rhythms and leave jet lag lagging behind. Of course, the best way to avoid jet lag is to fly north-south, rather than east–west: So how about exploring the possibilities of sticking to your own longitude?

51

Animal magic

We're used to seeing dogs leading the blind or assisting the deaf, but did you know pets can help nurse you back to health? Find out why this is no shaggy-dog story.

Pets bring fun to dull days, introduce you to new friends, and never tire of your voice.

They won't ditch you when times are tough and nobody seems to care. Instead, they offer friendship and pleasure that can help ward off sadness.

PUPPY LOVE

The Baystate Medical Center in Springfield, Massachusetts, has had a pet visiting program for almost a decade. Volunteers bring dogs and cats to visit seriously ill patients in intensive care. Nurses have observed that pet visits ease loneliness and decrease symptoms of depression.

TALK TO THE ANIMALS

Researchers in Los Angeles conducted one of the largest scientific studies into the health benefits of pet ownership. They surveyed over 1,800 gay and bisexual men with AIDS and discovered that those with close attachments to pets were significantly less likely to suffer from depression than men with AIDS who did not have a four-legged friend.

Here's an idea for you... **Make sure that owning a pet doesn't become a (depressing) burden. It's a big commitment. Pets offer warmth and company, but many have heavy-duty needs of their own. If you haven't the time or space for your own lifesaver on a lead, why not offer to dog walk at your local rescue shelter?**

HEALING HOUNDS

Professor Odendaal, a South African researcher, studied six depressed people. They all had a daily visit from a dog lasting half an hour. Before the study, all six had low blood levels of chemicals responsible for creating feelings of enjoyment and happiness. After meeting the dogs, levels of these key chemicals increased in their bloodstreams. More importantly, they felt happier, too.

These top ten benefits of pet ownership will make you paws for thought:

1. No matter if it's a lizard or a llama, pets prevent isolation.
2. Caring for a four-legged friend gives your life meaning and reduces the aching emptiness common in depression.
3. Pets need you. They offer you a sense of being wanted when you feel the world's against you.
4. Walking the dog widens most people's circle of friends.
5. Animals make you more active, which helps depression in its own right.
6. Pets offer companionship and nonjudgmental affection.
7. Stroking furry animals relieves stress by lowering your blood pressure and pulse rate.
8. Pets give you something to nurture and care for.
9. Nurturing a pet has the effect of making you more attentive to your personal care and appearance
10. There's evidence that pet owners are less susceptible to stress and less likely to kill themselves.

FELINE GOOD

It's said the world is divided into cat lovers and dog lovers. Cat lovers enjoy watching the feisty independence of these little animals who have never become truly domesticated. Stroking cats lowers stress levels, but if yours is no lap cat, there's still a lot you can learn from her. Cats provide living examples of get up and go, stretching regularly to prevent stress, walking away from trouble, and, if you've ever seen one with a mouse, you'll know they never give up.

FISH TALES

You needn't miss out on the therapeutic benefits of pet ownership just because you live in a small space. Underwater life is engaging and soothing. Dental waiting room designers have long known that watching the fluid movement of fish ambling around an aquarium can relieve stress and helps you relax.

Walking a dog is great exercise. Discover how getting physical can help you beat the blues in IDEA 40, *Pedal pushers*.

Try another idea...

"To his dog, every man is Napoleon; hence the constant popularity of dogs."
ALDOUS HUXLEY

Defining idea...

"I never married because there was no need. I have three pets at home which answer the same purpose as a husband. I have a dog which growls every morning, a parrot which swears all afternoon, and a cat that comes home late at night."
MARIE CORELLI, novelist

Defining idea...

Q **My teenage son has been depressed after relentless bullying. As he now finds it quite hard to trust people and make new friends, his father and I have been thinking about getting him a puppy. He likes animals and is a responsible kid, but we don't want it to become a burden on him and stress him out with extra responsibility. What's your advice?**

A *Pets have helped people of all ages get over depression. Your son needs to be well enough for the intensive work necessary for looking after a puppy, otherwise your worries about overburdening him might turn out to be true. Have you thought about getting an older dog from a rescue home? Nurturing a special friend like this may give him the boost he needs, without the extra burdens that come with puppies. Before you rush out to the pet shop or dogs' home, speaking to your son about what he'd find most helpful will go a long way toward ensuring you make the right decision.*

Q **I live in an apartment building where animals are not allowed. One of my neighbors is partially sighted and is allowed to have a guide dog. Do you think I would be able to have a dog as therapy for my depression?**

A *This is a tricky one. Therapy dogs aren't generally recognized in the way that guide dogs for the blind are. There are cases where people have taken their local authority or landlord to court, claiming that their pet is essential to their well-being, but this can be a long and painful process. I don't know your circumstances, but it might be easier to find somewhere else to live.*

52

The future's bright

Like a trusted old friend, depression is likely to come back from time to time. Learn how to show dark moods the door and shut out relapses.

Unfortunately, once depression has paid you a visit, it's likely to return. The good news is that you can send it packing, as long as you recognize its calling card.

Do you worry how you'll cope in the future? Many people wonder how they'll manage after stopping drugs or therapy.

Here's how. Think back to when you became depressed:

- What was going on at the time?
- What were you feeling?
- What sorts of things were you thinking about?
- Did you do anything differently?
- How long were things like this before you became depressed?
- With hindsight, what was the first thing you noticed was different?

Here's an idea for you...

If you're having trouble recognizing the early warning signs of your depression, try casting your mind back to when you became depressed and asking yourself the following questions: Did you lose interest in stuff you used to enjoy? Were you waking earlier than usual and finding you couldn't get back to sleep? Did you stop eating? Did anyone notice that you acted differently around other people? In what way?

If you're finding it difficult to recognize any warning signs, why not recruit some help? People you live with are often good at noticing subtle signs, but friends can be a good bet, too. Once you can recognize depression's forewarning, you're able to stop it in its tracks. These signs vary widely. Elliot, who usually struggles to get up, starts waking up early. Janine, a real foodie, loses interest in cooking and her appetite dwindles. For some people it's much more vague. Hilda feels "not right" but finds it hard to put into words. No problem with that, as long as she knows what it means and, more importantly, what she needs to do about it.

Think ahead over the next year and identify any events that are likely to trigger depression. Maybe your daughter is leaving home or your dad is getting very frail. It doesn't have to be anything major, and for many people it might be post-holiday blues. You might not be able to avoid events that could set off depression, like moving house or having a baby, but at least you can plan around them. Once you've identified potentially tricky times, I'm going to ask you to do something that can be daunting. I'd like you to imagine your depression has come back. Maybe your relationship has broken up, or you've lost your home or job. Using your answers to the following questions, come up with a battle plan:

- How will you deal with depression when it returns?
- What have you learned from previous episodes?

- What helped you get better?
- What ideas will you use now?
- What lines of attack are unhelpful?
- What could be done if it happened now?
- What would lessen its impact?
- Who else can help you?

Being depressed doesn't have to stop you from doing anything you set your mind to. Be inspired by the greats in IDEA 1, *Look to the stars.*

Try another idea...

It's a good idea to jot your answers down. They're a kind of first-aid kit to keep the initial flush of sadness away. Some people like to keep them wherever they keep bandages, painkillers, and other medical supplies. Why not add some emergency numbers to it, like your doctor, any pros you're seeing, any friends who are helpful in crises, and your local emergency department?

CALL IN REINFORCEMENTS

Seeing supportive friends and family can be key to defeating depression. You can divvy up responsibilities and be helped with overwhelming tasks. Inevitably, you'll think back to the last time you were depressed, but instead of dwelling on how terrible things are, try to consider what helped you feel better last time. If you can keep some sort of routine going, so much the better.

"I like living. I have sometimes been wildly, despairingly, acutely miserable, racked with sorrow, but through it all I still know that just to be alive is a grand thing."
AGATHA CHRISTIE

Defining idea...

And finally, consider:

- What have you learned that has worked for you?
- What can you do to build on what you've learned?

How did it go?

Q **I was seriously depressed earlier this year. Thankfully, I'm over it now. Will it definitely come back?**

A   *No. You may well be one of the 50 percent of people who become depressed and never get it again. In part, it depends how old you are. The older you are when you get depressed, the more likely it is to come back. Unfortunately, once it's back, it's more likely to make repeat appearances. The more times you get depression, the more likely you are to get it again.*

Q **My mom has had two bad bouts of depression. If it happens again, will it always be as bad?**

A   *Not necessarily. Encourage your mom to learn about her depression. Having had it twice, she'll already be able to recognize early warning signs and start using her favorite tricks to defeat it, as well as getting professional help if she needs it.*

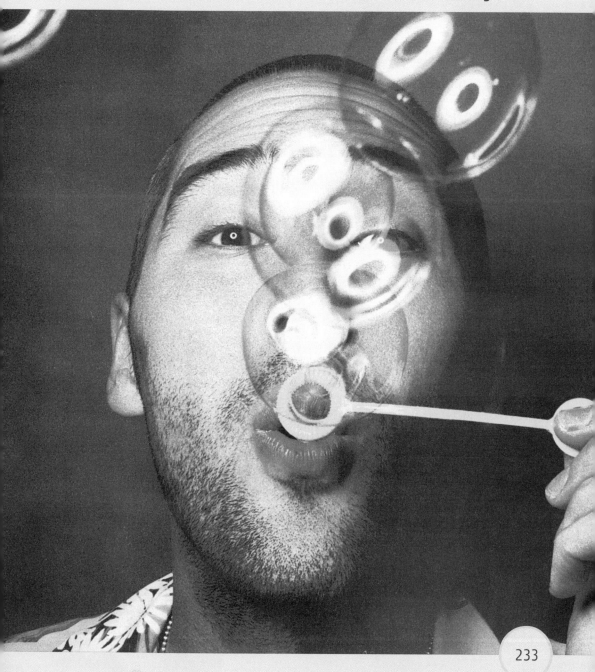

233

Where it's at...